Sexual Consequences
of Disability

SEXUAL CONSEQUENCES
OF DISABILITY

EDITED BY

ALEX COMFORT, M.B., Ph.D., D.Sc.

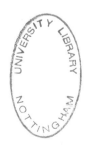

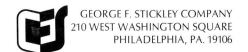
GEORGE F. STICKLEY COMPANY
210 WEST WASHINGTON SQUARE
PHILADELPHIA, PA. 19106

Acknowledgments

The Physiology of Human Penile Erection was reprinted by permission of the Annals of Internal Medicine, Volume 76: 793–799, 1972. The Handicapped and Sexual Health was reprinted by permission from SIECUS Report, Vol. IV, May, 1976. Sexual Impotence and Some Autonomic Disturbances in Men with Multiple Sclerosis was reprinted by permission from Acta Neurologica Scandinavica, Volume 45: 166–182, 1969. Sexual Dysfunction in Diabetic Men was reprinted by permission from Diabetes, Volume 23, 1974.

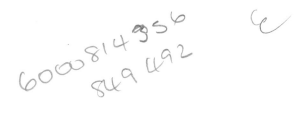

Manufactured in the United States of America; Published by the George F. Stickley Company, 210 W. Washington Square, Philadelphia, PA. 19106.

Contributors

Donald M. Barnett, M.D., Physician, Joslin Clinic, Boston, Massachusetts; Coordinator, Professional Resources, Diabetic Treatment Unit, New England Deaconess Hospital, Boston; and Instructor in Medicine, Harvard Medical School.

Rose Boyarsky, Ph.D., Research Associate in Urology, Division of Urology, Washington University; and President, Boyhill Center for Psychological Services, St. Louis, Missouri.

Saul Boyarsky, M.D., Professor of Urologic Surgery, Division of Urology, and Professor of Bioengineering, Washington University, St. Louis, Missouri.

Sandra S. Cole, B.A., Coordinator, Physical Disabilities Section Program in Human Sexuality, University of Minnesota Medical School, Minneapolis, Minnesota.

Theodore M. Cole, M.D., Professor of Physical Medicine and Rehabilitation, University of Minnesota Medical School, Minneapolis, Minnesota.

Alex Comfort, M.B., B.Ch. (Cantab.), M.R.C.S., L.R.C.P., D.C.H., Ph.D., D.Sc. (London). Fellow, Institute for Higher Studies, Santa Barbara, California; Consultant, Geriatric Psychiatry, Brentwood V.A. Hospital; Clinical Lecturer, Department of Psychiatry, Stanford University; Associate Professor, Department of Psychiatry, U.S.C.

Roger T. Crenshaw, M.D., The Crenshaw Clinic, Hillcrest North Medical Center, San Diego, California.

Theresa L. Crenshaw, M.D., The Crenshaw Clinic, San Diego, California.

Mona M. Devanesan, M.D., Associate Professor, Department of Obstetrics and Gynecology, New Jersey College of Medicine (CMDNJ), Newark, New Jersey.

George E. Ehrlich, M.D., Director, The Arthritis Center, Albert Einstein Medical Center and Moss Rehabilitation Hospital, Philadelphia, Pennsylvania.

William L. Furlow, M.D., Department of Urology, Mayo Clinic, and Associate Professor of Urology, Mayo Medical School, Rochester, Minnesota.

H. Howard Goldstein, M.D., Staff Physician, New England Deaconess Hospital, Boston, Massachusetts; and Assistant Clinical Professor of Medicine, Harvard Medical School.

Cecily Green, Adjunct Sex Therapist, Center for Social and Sensory Learning, Los Angeles, California.

Lauro S. Halstead, M.D., Texas Institute for Rehabilitation and Research, Texas Medical Center, Houston, Texas.

Charles B. Kahn, M.D., Clinical Assistant Professor of Medicine, Brown Program in Medicine, Brown University, Providence, Rhode Island.

Contributors

Robert C. Kolodny, M.D., Associate Director of Reproductive Biology Research Foundation, St. Louis, Missouri; Head of Endocrinological Research.

Norman B. Levy, M.D., Associate Professor, Department of Psychiatry, Downstate Medical Center, Brooklyn, New York.

Francis G. Mackey, M.D., Medical Director, St. Jude Hospital and Rehabilitation Center, Fullerton, California.

Joanne E. Mantell, M.S.S.W., M.S.P.H., UCLA School of Public Health, Division of Behavioral Sciences and Health Education, Los Angeles, California.

David E. Martin, Ph.D., Yerkes Regional Primate Research Center of Emory University, and College of Allied Health Sciences, Georgia State University, Atlanta, Georgia.

Dennis J. Massler, M.D., Clinical Assistant Professor, Departments of Obstetrics, Gynecology, and Psychiatry, New Jersey College of Medicine (CMDNJ), Newark, New Jersey.

Domeena C. Renshaw, M.D., Professor, Department of Psychiatry, Loyola University Medical Center, Maywood, Illinois.

Margaret E. Symonds, M.D., Medical Director, Children's Specialized Hospital, Westfield, New Jersey; Assistant Clinical Professor in Pediatrics, Columbia University College of Physicians and Surgeons, New York.

C.J. Vas, M.B., Department of Neurology, The General Infirmary, Leeds 1, Yorkshire, England.

Harold Warner, Yerkes Regional Primate Research Center of Emory University, Atlanta, Georgia.

Howard D. Weiss, M.D., Department of Medicine, Rush-Presbyterian-St. Luke's Medical Center, and Northwestern University Medical School, Chicago, Illinois.

Loraine D. Wickware, R.N., E.T., Director, Stoma Rehabilitation Clinic, Children's Specialized Hospital, Westfield, New Jersey.

Contents

Contents

Introduction

Physicians are aware that the valuation of sexuality in our culture has undergone, and is still undergoing, a change. This change is less a *sexual revolution* in the behavioral sense than a general increase in frankness and expectation. Among those who are affected by these changes are patients whose disorder, or the medication we prescribe for it, affects their sexual functioning, and the *disabled*—persons with irremediable or progressive loss of sensory or motor function.

Patients whose illness affects their sex life—even if it is only a transient infection, such as trichomoniasis, or a recurrent nuisance, such as bladder infection in women—now volunteer interference with intercourse as a primary symptom. Iatrogenic impotence produced by antihypertensive drugs, for example, which was formerly a cause of silent noncompliance, is now recognized and complained of by patients. With the recognition that sexual function is normally lifelong, needlessly radical prostatic surgery compromising potency or pelvic surgery compromising intercourse has become proper grounds for a malpractice suit. Clearly the conspiracy of silence which formerly existed between doctor and patient over sexuality—to be broken only in vague generalities—is at an end, and coital function and satisfaction have to be confronted on the same terms as mobility and the enjoyment of food as part of the "quality of life." While most physicians would welcome this development as healthy, the traditional reticences have left a legacy: sex counseling was not taught in medical schools until recently, and so far not a single medical textbook has been published in which the specifically sexual effects of common diseases could be looked up. If the patient in whom we diagnose amyotrophic lateral sclerosis asks us, "Will it affect my sex life?" it would take most of us a literature search to reply.

In the case of people whom society labels as disabled, whether their disorder is congenital, idiopathic, or the result of accident, both we and they are liable to find ourselves the victims of social "black magic." The negative attitude of most persons toward the disabled, the unconscious castration anxieties which disability or deformity excite, and the real social problems of sexual expression in isolated or institutionalized people are often dealt with by projection: the sexual needs of such people are better minimized or ignored, rather than discussed, for fear of embarrassing them—by which we mean that they embarrass or disturb us. Their sexual needs attract the same disapproval we accord to the sexual needs of older persons, as though they were in some way unseemly.

GENDER IDENTITY

Of all the body image perceptions which contribute to ego-security and to a robust sense of personhood, functioning gender identity as an acceptable, desirable and sexual man or woman is among the most important. For those whose other modes of personal reinforcement are compromised by motor defects, dependency and isolation, sexuality becomes not less but *more* significant as an assertion of personal worth and a source of physical and mental satisfaction. Attempts of those around them to pretend that these needs do not exist, to condemn their manifestation, and to divert the patient's attention (for his or her own good, of course) into substitute channels like chess and CB radio are always questionable. And with the growing and sometimes excessive public expectation today in the field of sexuality, they are becoming untenable. The general style of the culture does not stop at the door of the disabled person's room, or at the perimeter of an institution. The newly disabled patient whose first question is "Will I be able to walk?" now asks a second question, "What will this do to my sex life?" and seeks intelligent prognosis, discussion and rehabilitation in both areas.

When we attempt to address this problem, we find that the "disabled" person has two types of disabilities to contend with in the sexual field: those arising from physical problems which limit activity or response, and those arising from misinformation and lack of social permission. It is the second of these, which the disabled share with the able, which accounts for the major part of the difficulty. Folklore regards sexual activity as "performance" (a damaging misconception which underlies almost all psychogenic sexual dysfunction and which can be aggravated by replacing guilt and anxiety over sex with unrealistic expectations). It is focused exclusively on the genitalia—sex means putting an erect penis in a receptive vagina, and any other type of activity is at best preparatory or substitutional and at worst *abnormal* or deviant. Physicians repeatedly see patients whose sole disability is limitation of movement in a hip joint and who complain that intercourse is painful or impossible because they believe that it can properly be undertaken in only one position. Males who for organic reasons are unable to obtain full, or any, erection very commonly believe themselves to be incapable of intercourse and even incapable of obtaining satisfaction or giving it to a partner... all of these beliefs are without factual basis. Moralistic and early psychoanalytic interpretations of nongenital sexual techniques retain much force in attitude and folklore even when patients pay lip service to their normality in man and their generality in mammals; they may be *all right* but they are not *the real thing.*

The need for more realistic sex counseling which recognizes sexual expression as something involving the whole body and the whole person, undertaken for relationship and mutual pleasure and not as a demonstration, is constantly seen in the able. Problems in this area are self-aggravating: it is normal, for example, for the amount of tactile stimulation needed to produce erection and the latent period of full erection to increase with age, and orgasm not to occur at every act of intercourse. The male whose stereotype of sexual *performance* involves hurried erection with minimal preliminaries followed by equally hurried intercourse experiences these changes as *loss of virility* and may become functionally impotent through anxiety over them, while the more sexually educated male often welcomes them as an improvement in pleasure-potential. The patient who is incapable through limitation of movement or sensation of performing certain sexual acts may react in the same way—he or she has a prospectus of what sexual adequacy should be, and any failure to meet this program constitutes asexuality or dysfunction.

CULTURAL CONSTRUCTS

Besides the pressures of folklore, individuals whose mobility is limited or whose deformity is evident are exposed to other forms of attack upon their sense of worth and desirability. Cultural constructs, such as a wholly unrealistic emphasis on physical beauty or strength as an index of being desirable, and the practical barriers to finding a partner, all combine to make the aim of sexual self-validation seem better given up; the relief of hospital staff and relatives when this renunciation becomes evident may contribute to it, even though they do nothing to remedy the frustration and loss of self-value which may accompany it. It was my practice at one time to keep a roster of double amputees who danced, swam and rode bicycles to visit and reassure those faced with this type of surgery. For a disabled person, conversation with an equally handicapped or disfigured individual who is functioning fully with a valuing and affectionate partner is one of the best forms of therapy, but it obviously does not remove the practical difficulties of partner-search. Its function is to widen inner options by making evident the following facts: that no person is incapable through physical infirmity of giving and exciting caring affection in another, based on valuation and not pity or any other dependency-inducing emotion; that relatively few people are incapable of mutually satisfying intercourse, or a rewarding substitute for it; that no one is without sexual needs, physical and sociopsychological, through physical infirmity alone; and that even if for other reasons overt sexual expression is renounced or is infrequent by deliberate choice on practical grounds, the knowledge of our capacity for it and the reality of the option is a necessary part of healthy self-esteem.

AIMS AND OBJECTIVES

In this book we have attempted to address the problems of information concerning the sexual effects of common disorders, as well as the question of sex and disability. The first of these is necessary if we are to practice intelligently in the modern climate of public expectation. In regard to the second, if we are still anxious and fear that the ill-effects of overzealous interference may disturb or be seen as impertinent, this can only mean that we have not communicated frankly with disabled adults. They have no such doubts. On the other hand, a great many are discouraged, uncertain where to turn for counseling, and inclined to "do as the man says" to avoid unpleasantness in a setting where their dependency on others is already onerous. Some need their general attitude to sexuality to be restructured by permission, exactly as do many able individuals: some will react to this restructuring with anxiety, as do many able individuals. But for most, the realization that many who consider themselves sexually disabled are nothing of the kind, and owe their concept of sexual adequacy to folklore and role-playing, is extremely reinforcing. This is an area where the restoration or establishment of function—or even of the awareness that function is possible—can produce massive beneficial effects in all areas.

The heavy emphasis in the succeeding chapters on male problems is a consequence of our culture. Not only does male sexual expression involve the outward and visible sign of an inner and spiritual grace, but its perception in patients both able and disabled is performance-loaded, and this bias is reflected in all of the available research data. For example, it is easy to document the effect of drugs on male but not on female sexual physiology. If we have failed to redress this balance, that is simply because data are often lacking. The only possible excuse for this performance-orientation in the literature to date is that female paraplegics, for example, adjust more easily than do males to the attainment of extragenital orgasm. On the other hand, the growing problem of mastectomy• is addressed in special sections of the book, together with the issues raised by pelvic surgery.

Broad issues of institutional policy regarding patients with sexual problems are not discussed fully in this book. Its aim is to provide physicians with a series of reviews covering a number of the less familiar areas of sexual counseling in relation to disease, disability and medication. Though not entirely comprehensive, it may prove helpful in orienting the physician in office practice to the subject of sexual medicine, and it is with this objective that the topics included have been selected.

1

Sex Counseling of the Disabled
in Medical Practice

ALEX COMFORT, M.B.

Much work is now in progress in counseling disabled people with sexual problems. It is desultory, however, and the needs of patients with various disabilities, as well as the range and efficacy of specific advice to be given, have never been documented fully. This lack is important, since much of the necessary counseling could be done in family practice, especially if conditions such as mastectomy are included in the range of disabilities. Most published material has concentrated on spinal injury, where the sexual problems are of a special kind. Those of spastic paralysis, rheumatoid and other arthritis, multiple sclerosis and most other chronic disabling disorders are quite inadequately documented.

It is important to realize that sexual anxiety and sexual dysfunction are extremely common in the general population—the disabled contend with these psychosocial influences as well as with the special problems of their disability. The general physician will probably have to deal with cases where intercurrent illness, medication or surgery upsets an established sexual adjustment. He requires close familiarity with the psychosexual implications of common drugs such as antihypertensives, common disorders (diabetes, heart disease), common surgical interventions (mastectomy, prostatectomy) and a general awareness of those involved in spinal injury, for instance. In regard to medication, inquiry into and knowledge of pharmacological effects on sexual response is an important part of prescribing: the alternatives are noncompliance, or compliance with serious injury to the quality of life, as in the uncomplaining hypertensive who has become needlessly impotent. The effect of medication on sexuality in women is a yawning gap in our knowledge—one which only systematic inquiry by prescribers can fill.

All surgery involves some assault on the body image, and the psychosexual consequences will be proportionate to the extent of the threat. While this is obvious in the case of mastectomy, amputation or disfigurement, it is equally true that oophorectomy or hysterectomy performed without adequate patient explanation and reassurance amounts to incomplete or negligent surgery. If the surgeon himself communicates most comfortably with the anesthetized patient, he must delegate the important task of exploring patient anxiety to a colleague who may well be the family physician. In Britain, for example, it is with the family practitioner that the options, and advice of the surgical consultant, will be explored in a psychotherapeutic milieu. The special case of prostatectomy presents great difficulty because of the uncertainty of the functional result: some individuals retain potency after widespread surgery, while others are seriously disabled by minimal transurethral resection. On one hand, retention of function correlates highly with previous sexual satisfaction and loss of function with performance anxiety. On the other hand, alteration of ejaculatory sensation may be unavoidable. Moreover, in fracture of the pelvis, impotency correlates highly with urethral injury (King 1975) for reasons which are unclear. Transurethral prostatectomy which appears to avoid injury to critical structures may in fact act in the same manner.

Surgery which involves the genitalia and pelvic organs, which interrupts reflex arcs, which involves radiation exposure to the pelvis, or which combines such direct anatomical impairment with an "unesthetic" or confidence-reducing result (cystostomy, colostomy) can be mitigated by prior education, sexual counseling, and the assistance of patient groups. Major injury to the central nervous system, especially paraplegia, is a special case, and the management of its sexual implications is particularly well-documented. The chapters included in this book have been deliberately chosen to address other areas less well-documented, which the physician who is conscious of the psychosexual dimension will have to deal with constantly—post-coronary heart disease and cerebrovascular accident rehabilitation, arthritis, diabetes and other common conditions. In all of these, the pattern of management is the same:

   1) *Ascertain the exact extent of the physical problem.* If erection is impaired, examine by plethysmography or nocturnal tumescence recording whether response is really absent,

or is secondarily inhibited. If orgasm has been lost, compare with the pre-morbid history, inquire into changes in sexual practice and self-estimate. If movement is impaired, precisely what movements are lost? Simple or unanalyzed complaints of "no erection" or "no satisfaction" must be tactfully dissected: thus anorgasmia may in fact represent dyspnea at one extreme or feelings of disfigurement and rejection at the other.

2) *Widen the sexual repertoire* by education and permission. If coitus is impossible in the habitual position, encourage use of others. If intromission is impossible, educate the couple in the use and propriety of extragenital techniques. If genital sensation is impaired, encourage the search for extragenital sensation. Although for some couples this may appear to involve a complete sexual re-education too extensive for the busy physician, a great deal of good (or harm) can be done by a few words and by the attitude of the counselor. The physician must be constantly vigilant to avoid *bewitching* a patient by unguarded warnings or *obiter dicta*. If he cannot project a positive attitude towards sexuality, or deal with his own social background and countertransference, he should refer to a qualified sex therapist.

3) *Set goals* both for the patient undergoing rehabilitation and for the disabled patient developing sexual skills. Rather than making sexuality a subject of anxious performance-testing, suggest a model in which it is the task of the couple and the physician to devise means of outwitting the disease or the limitation. In this context one observes repeatedly that people whose sexuality prior to disability was functional but perfunctory can actually, properly counseled, use the adverse circumstance as a stimulus to overcome earlier rigidity and haste.

How much counseling the individual physician cares to undertake is a matter of time and taste. On the other hand, it is not possible to practice medicine or surgery at all in areas which impinge on sexual functioning without entering the area of psychotherapy and doing either good or harm there. Information on the practicalities of sexual dysfunction is a starting minimum. Beyond that, the success we have in helping patients deal with the problems of their sexuality, whether general or special, will depend very often on how well we have dealt with our own.

COMMONLY SEEN PROBLEMS

The problems of sex and disability most commonly seen in office practice are not those associated with paraplegias or major systemic diseases. They are:

   1) interference with habitual sexual behavior by a relatively minor disability (arthritis, asthma), or by side-effects of medication;
   2) convalescence from coronary heart disease;
   3) sequelae of common surgical procedures (mastectomy, prostatectomy).

"Habitual sexual behavior" means the pattern to which the patient has become accustomed—even a change of venue can disrupt the relaxation necessary for sexual function in some people. The pattern may cover rigid and mistaken beliefs about normality—patients who say they "cannot have intercourse" may mean only that it is no longer possible in the male-superior position. Or a man accustomed to hasty sexual intercourse may describe himself as impotent because arousal now takes longer. In all of these common presentations, counseling is the major part of therapy, and involves sexual education.

Major disabilities require special advice. *Lower limb amputees* are seldom sexually at a disadvantage, though they may suffer through self-consciousness. The physician should be aware that amputation in itself has psychosymbolic overtones for some individuals, however, and that an amputated partner may exercise a fetishistic attraction. *Exercise-induced bronchial asthma* can be sexually disabling. Symington and Kerr (1976) found that this problem could be elicited in many asthmatics, but was rarely volunteered. The hyperventilation of intercourse, anxiety, and the stirring-up of bed dust containing house-mite debris all probably contribute. It responds well to prophylactic treatment.

Of accidental injuries short of damage to the genitalia and central nervous system, only severe crush injuries and fracture of the pelvis commonly lead to organic impotence. In pelvic fractures, impotence correlates with involvement of the urethra, for reasons not fully clear. In many cases the cessation of intercourse after the accident leads to a secondary psychologic impotence due to performance anxiety—if therapy and rehabilitation are directed to this early in convalescence, the mischief can be avoided (King 1975).

If physicians recognize that early resexualization is as important as early ambulation, and inquire diligently and tactfully into the sexual adaptation of patients, they can perform important therapy in limiting unnecessary dysfunction, and equally important research in detecting other common and remediable psychosexual problems of illness which their patients have been suffering in silence. Sexually unanxious patients overcome paralysis, high-injury disorders such as hemophilia and osteogenesis imperfecta, and indeed, practically all but the most incapacitating diseases. In a few major diseases, moreover, reassurance on this score can be given: amyotrophic lateral sclerosis is a case in point, since sexual function, at least in males, persists even in the presence of terminal motor paralysis (Jokelainen and Palo 1976). In both diabetes and post-prostatectomy, physical impairment may be grossly compounded by anxiety and anxiety mistaken for organic impotence.

It is a safe assumption that in all relevant illness, sexuality is involved along with other life activities; that counseling and inquiry are part of the structure of specific treatment; and that the physician should consider sexual rehabilitation and the prophylaxis of bewitchment exactly as he considers occupational rehabilitation, but perhaps with even greater urgency. Now that both patient and counselor are more able than in the past to take the examination of sexuality in their stride, much needless dysfunction can be avoided.

REFERENCES

JOKELAINEN, M. and PALO, J. Amyotrophic lateral sclerosis and the nervous system. Lancet 1:1246, 1976.

KING, J. Impotence after fractures of the pelvis. J. Bone Joint Surg. 57A:1107-9, 1975.

SYMINGTON, I. and KERR, J.W. Sexercise-induced asthma. Lancet 2:693, 1976.

2

The Physiology of
Human Penile Erection

HOWARD D. WEISS, M.D.

The study of human penile erection and its disorders has not been completely adopted by specialists in any particular medical discipline, although the subject is closely related to urology, neurology, psychiatry, and internal medicine. Consequently, relatively few physicians have a basic understanding of the physiology of penile erection—knowledge that is essential to formulate a logical approach to the patients' problems. This chapter summarizes current concepts of the neurological and hemodynamic mechanisms mediating human penile erection, using them to explain the common causes of erectile dysfunction.

STIMULI FOR ERECTION

Penile erection is a reflex phenomenon over which man has little direct voluntary control, that is, man cannot will or demand an erection.[1] The forms of stimulation that can reflexly elicit erection have been classified as either "psychogenic" or "reflexogenic." Auditory, visual, olfactory, gustatory, tactile, and imaginative stimuli may arouse the erotic centers of the brain and result in a so-called "psychogenic erection." Exteroceptive stimulation of the genital regions (for example, lightly stroking the glans penis) or vague interoceptive stimuli arising in the bladder or rectum may produce a so-called "reflexogenic erection."[2] Interoceptive impulses cause seemingly spontaneous erections, since man is not consciously aware of these visceral signals. More than 70 per cent of the erections occurring during sleep have been associated with the dream phase.[3] Many of these erections are probably psychogenic in origin; the remainder are reflex responses to visceral or tactile impulses.

Psychic and reflexogenic stimuli often act synergistically in producing erections. For example, in a normal man the degree of tactile genital stimulation required to produce erection is diminished in the presence of concomitant erotic psychic stimulation. Intero- and extero-ceptive stimulation may also act synergistically; in normal man reflexogenic erections occur more readily when the bladder is full than when the bladder is empty. Also, psychogenic stimuli such as guilt or hostility, often acting at a subconscious level, can inhibit the erection reflex. The ability of local extero- and intero-ceptive stimuli to inhibit erections is less clear, although urologists have used local nociceptive stimuli to prevent erections during operative procedures.

NEUROPHYSIOLOGY OF ERECTION

Experimentation on the neurophysiology of erection began more than 100 years ago, when Eckhardt[4] reported that electrical stimulation of the visceral (parasympathetic) branches of nerves from the sacral spinal cord produced penile erection in dogs. He called these nerves the "nervi erigentes" (erigentes being the Latin term for erection). Electrical stimulation of the pudendal nerve (a somatic nerve from the sacral cord segments) did not cause erection, but destruction of the pudendal nerve abolished the dog's erectile response to mechanical stimulation of the penis.[5] This suggested that the pudendal nerves carried the afferent impulses necessary for reflexogenic erections. Semans and Langworthy's[6] famous experiments on cats later produced similar observations.

In man, efferent neural impulses for erection are thought to arise from parasympathetic fibers in sacral cord roots S 2, S 3, and S 4, although recently the role of S 2 has been questioned.[7] These are the same spinal roots that provide the efferent (parasympathetic) supply to the detrusor muscle of the urinary bladder and to the distal colon and rectum. Thus the pelvic nerves from the sacral cord segments conduct the parasympathetic impulses for erection, micturition, and defecation. Men with partial spinal cord injuries but intact pelvic nerves frequently have a dissociation of bladder, bowel, and erectile function (for example, normal bladder and bowels with absent reflexogenic erections). Similarly, damage to the nerves in the pelvis may alter one of these physiologic functions without affecting the others. This shows that, although anatomically similar, these pathways are not identical. The usual decreasing order of vulnerability for these pathways is erection, bladder, and then bowel function.[8]

It is now evident, however, that pathways originating above the sacral cord level may also play a role in initiating erection. Root and Bard[9] removed the entire sacral spinal cord from male cats and found that in the presence of females in estrus, full penile erections would still occur. Conversely, manipulation of the penis of these cats would not produce an erection. When a second spinal cord transection was later made in the lower thoracic cord, the animals still showed signs of sexual excitement, such as attempted mounting, when placed with an estrous female, but no erections occurred. Combining destruction of the sacral cord with thoracolumbar sympathectomy also resulted in sexual excitement without any erections. These experiments suggest that a spinal outflow traveling via sympathetic pathways and requiring intact communication with higher centers can mediate psychogenic erections in the absence of the sacral spinal cord.

Similar observations have also been made in man. In a patient with an injury at the level of the first lumbar vertebra, it was therapeutically necessary to sever all anterior and posterior spinal roots below L 1. In this man the entire pelvic region had been denervated, and reflexogenic erections could not be elicited. Nevertheless, the patient still had erections associated with erotic psychic stimuli.[10]

The studies of Bors and Comarr[2] and of others[11-13] on men who have suffered spinal cord injuries have clarified the neuroanatomy of the spinal centers for erection. More than 90 per cent of patients with complete spinal cord transections located well above the sacral cord level were able to have erections, but these erections occurred only after reflexogenic stimuli and not after psychogenic stimuli. This indicates that, in the absence of suprasegmental connections, reflexogenic erections can occur entirely on the basis of sacral reflex. Bilateral pudendal nerve destruction should result in complete impotence in these cases since this eliminates the afferent limb of the reflex arc.[14] Conversely, about one-fourth of patients who suffered complete lower motor neuron lesions of the sacral cord were able to have erections after psychogenic stimuli but not after reflexogenic stimuli.[2] In patients with incomplete spinal cord lesions both psychogenic and reflexogenic erections may occur. These data suggest that an outflow from the thoracolumbar cord (estimated to originate around T 12-L 1) can mediate psychogenic erections in patients with complete sacral cord destruction.

Bilateral removal of all the sympathetic nerve chains below the diaphragm does not alter the erectile responses of male cats to females in estrus.[9] Since this procedure presumably destroys the efferent fibers from the thoracolumbar erection center, it indicates that in cats with intact spinal cords the sacral (parasympathetic) outflow is capable of mediating both psychogenic and reflexogenic erections. Rose[15] did not report any disturbances in erection after bilateral lumbar sympathectomy in 30 men or bilateral thoracolumbar sympathectomy in 8 men. Whitelaw and Smithwick[16] found that 26 of 112 men suffered a "disturbance of erection" after undergoing bilateral thoracolumbar sympathectomy. Unfortunately, they did not specify the degree of erectile dysfunction (partial or complete) or whether reflexogenic or psychogenic erections selectively occurred in individual cases. At present, bilateral sympathectomy has not been shown to have any consistent effect on erectile function in man.

A logical interpretation of the various observations is that an outflow from the thoracolumbar cord acts synergistically with the sacral parasympathetic outflow to mediate penile erections. The sacral erection center receives reflex-arc input from both local reflexogenic stimuli (mainly via the pudendal nerves) and from psychic stimuli originating in the higher centers of the central nervous system. The thoracolumbar erection center receives reflex-arc input from the higher centers but not directly from reflexogenic stimuli. Autonomic nerves from the thoracolumbar (sympathetic) outflow have been found to contain both vasoconstrictor (adrenergic) and vasodilator (cholinergic) fibers.[17] The failure of direct electrical stimulation of these nerves to produce penile erection may be attributed to simultaneous stimulation of the antagonistic fibers. Presumably an erection-mediating (vasodilator) component is selectively activated by erotic psychic stimuli. In normal men it is difficult to assess the relative roles played by the thoracolumbar and sacral centers in producing erections, but it is clear that in cases of complete impotence the outflow from both centers must be compromised.

CEREBRAL REPRESENTATION OF ERECTION

Knowledge of the cerebral representation of penile erection comes mainly from experiments on monkeys.[18-21] MacLean[22] and his group have attempted to elicit penile erections and other sexual responses in the squirrel monkey by using stereotaxically placed electrodes to electrically stimulate cortical and brainstem structures. Considering the importance of sexual function for species survival, it is not surprising that most of the cerebral tissue from which electrical stimulation can evoke penile erections is related to the limbic system, phylogenetically the oldest part of the brain. The limbic system is understood to coordinate sensory inputs with visceral function and emotion in men and animals. Electrical stimulation in the lateral medial hypothalamus, the septal-preoptic region, or along the inferior thalamic peduncle was very effective in eliciting erection. In addition, erections were evoked by stimulating some points not in the limbic system, such as in the putamen.[21]

MacLean traced the major effector pathway for erection in monkeys from the septal area downward to a position just lateral to the pyramidal tracts at the junction of the pons and medulla.[22] The erection pathway passes through regions that contain limbic, extrapyramidal, and neocortical outflows, a fact that may provide the anatomical clue to the integration of these systems. The visceral efferent pathways connecting the brain with the thoracolumbar and sacral erection centers are thought to descend in the lateral columns of the spinal cord, in the vicinity of the pyramidal tracts.

There are relatively few reports dealing with cerebral localization of penile erections in humans, and consequently our knowledge is quite fragmentary. Meyers[23] reported two cases in which the ansa lenticularis was sectioned bilaterally to relieve myoclonus, with resultant postoperative impotence and loss of libido. The surgical lesions crossed areas analogous to regions in the monkey brain where electrical stimulation produces erections.[22] Stimulation of electrodes implanted in the septal region of the human brain leads to pleasurable sensations and, occasionally, penile erections,[24] as has been found in monkeys. Temporal lobe lesions in man have been associated with loss of erectile ability but normal libido.[25] Temporal lobectomy in man sometimes results in the inability to have erections, but this effect may be transient. Bilateral temporal lobectomy in man may result in hypersexuality and other behavior disorders[26] similar to those first described in monkeys by Klüver and Bucy.[27]

The possibility that a cerebral lesion can cause complete impotence is interesting from a theoretical point of view. The cerebral outflow is not absolutely necessary for erections to occur, as witnessed by the patients with complete spinal cord transections who continue to have erections. Therefore, if a cerebral lesion can produce complete impotence, we can speculate that the lesion might be depressing facilitory pathways to the spinal erection centers while leaving inhibitory pathways intact. The unbalanced inhibitory influence presumably causes the erectile dysfunction. Little is known about the physiologic mechanisms and anatomic pathways that mediate cerebral inhibition of erection, although this information would be of great importance in understanding how psychological factors cause impotence.

HEMODYNAMICS OF ERECTION

The actual transformation of the penis from a flaccid to an erect state is a vascular phenomenon. Blood reaches the penis via terminal branches of the right and left internal pudendal arteries. These vessels carry blood to the "erectile tissues" of the penis: two corpora cavernosa lying side by side on the dorsal aspect of the penis and the corpus spongiosum surrounding the urethra. The erectile tissues consist of irregular sponge-like systems of vascular spaces interspersed between the arteries and veins.[28] When the penis is flaccid, the vascular spaces contain very little blood and are virtually collapsed. During erection the vascular spaces are transformed into large cavities distended with blood at high pressures.[29]

The distention of the penis with blood during erection is brought about by the opening of anastomoses between the arterioles and the vascular spaces in the erectile tissues. Conti[30] carefully studied the vascular morphology of the human penis and concluded that there are valve-like structures called "polsters" containing smooth muscle located at the anastomoses between the arterioles and the vascular spaces. The polsters cause blood to be shunted away from the corpora cavernosa directly into the veins when the penis is flaccid. The polsters are under the control of the autonomic nervous system (fibers from the sacral and thoracolumbar erection centers) and relax when impulses for erection are transmitted, thereby allowing a greatly increased volume of blood to flow into the vascular spaces of the erectile tissues.[31] The rate of arterial inflow is temporarily greater than the rate of venous outflow, thus causing the characteristic increase in penile volume during erection. A steady-state is eventually reached, where the rates of inflow and outflow are equal and the penis ceases to enlarge but remains rigid.[32]

These facts were nicely demonstrated in experiments on human volunteers and cadavers, in which it was shown that the rate of perfusion of the corpora cavernosa is correlated with the degree of penile distention.[31] Once erection was secured, however, it could be maintained by a somewhat slower flow. Animal experiments have also demonstrated the importance of continuous high-volume flow for erection. For example, mechanical constriction of the aorta during an erection will promptly cause the erection to subside.[6]

Polsters are also present in the erectile tissue drainage veins, thus leading to the speculation that these polsters contract when the arteriolar polsters dilate, thereby promoting turgescence by diminishing the venous outflow.[33] Newman et al.[31] believe that venous blockade is not necessary for human penile erection and probably does not occur. They found that occlusion of the venous return from the erectile tissues of ten human volunteers produced a cyanotic and edematous but not erect penis. Several investigators believe that erection also requires a decrease in blood flow to the somatic (nonerectile) tissues of the penis.[30,31]

Newman proposes that sympathetic nerve impulses might contribute to erection by constricting the arterioles in the penis that do not supply blood to the erectile tissues, but there is no experimental verification of such a mechanism.

Reflex contraction of the ischiocavernosus and bulbocavernosus muscles has been thought to pump blood to the penis and to help maintain erection by mechanically obstructing venous drainage from the penis.[34,35] Observations of humans[2,31] and animals[29,36,37] have shown that the ischio- and bulbocavernosus muscles do not play an essential role in penile erection. A brief contraction of these muscles may momentarily increase penile rigidity, but in fact patients with flaccid paralysis of all pelvic musculature can have completely normal erections.[2] Some passive venous obstruction undoubtedly occurs when the thin-walled vascular spaces in the distended corpora cavernosa are compressed against the thick fibrous membrane, the tunica albuginea, that surrounds each corpus cavernosum.[38] The corpus spongiosum is not surrounded by a rigid fibrous membrane, and this might explain why the corpus spongiosum never attains the same great rigidity as the corpus cavernosum.

DETUMESCENCE OF THE PENIS

The mechanism for subsidence of penile erection is not clearly understood. If the psychic or reflexogenic stimulus that elicited the erection is not adequately sustained over time, detumescence of the penis normally occurs within a few moments. It is not known whether this is merely owing to diminution of the cholinergic (vasodilator) impulses that open the polsters or whether an active vasoconstrictor impulse is also involved. It has been stated (but not proved) that when ejaculation takes place erection subsides promptly because the sympathetic impulses that facilitate emission of semen also cause constriction of the vessels supplying blood to the erectile tissues of the penis.[5] Persistence of such impulses after ejaculation might explain the well-known latency period between ejaculation and the ability to have another erection shortly thereafter. Potts has suggested that some cases of impotence could be due to this "sympathetic hyper-excitability."[39] Unfortunately the reports on sympathectomy and sexual function do not mention whether sympathectomy affects the rate at which penile erections subside.[15,16]

Priapism, the prolonged failure of an erection to subside in the absence of sexual stimulation, is frequently associated with certain hematologic disorders (for example, sickle-cell disease and chronic leukemias) but its cause may be unknown. The physiologic mechanism for priapism is poorly understood. In the hematologic cases priapism is thought to be related to occlusion of outflow from the penis by masses of irregular cells.[40] The idiopathic cases are believed to result from prolonged venous stasis with inflammation of the septa and edema. The edema supposedly obstructs the venous outflow, thereby promoting the priapism. The mechanism cannot be related to venous thrombosis, as the priapic penis is warm and red, not cyanotic or cold.[41] Priapism also occasionally occurs after acute spinal cord injuries, being commonest after cervical cord lesions.[12]

PHYSIOLOGIC EXPLANATIONS FOR IMPOTENCE

The pathways mediating human penile erection are schematically illustrated in Figure 1. The common causes of impotence can be explained physiologically by analyzing the underlying lesions in these pathways according to the diagram.

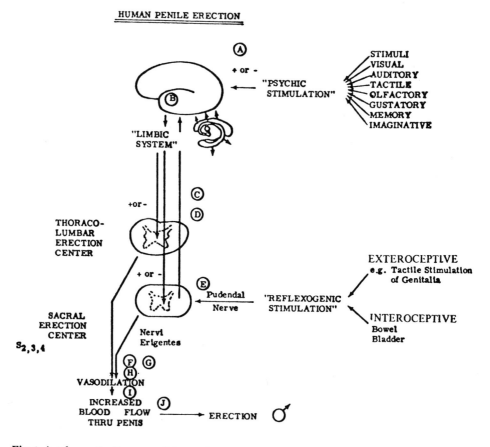

Fig. 1. A schematic diagram of the pathways involved in human penile erection, partially adapted from the illustrations of Semans and Langworthy[6] and Bors and Comarr.[2] The letters (A to J) represent potential sites of lesions that could cause erectile dysfunction.

SITE A

The ability of a given stimulus to cause penile erections in a normal man is greatly dependent on psychological factors, such as relaxation or fear, that may reinforce or completely inhibit the erection reflex.[1] Psychological factors are by far the commonest cause of erectile dysfunction in man. Some patients with complete psychic impotence will occasionally awaken in the morning with an erection, indicating that at least one of the spinal erection centers is intact and can function if released from suprasegmental inhibition. Unfortunately for the patient this release is initiated only during sleep. The physiologic mechanism and anatomic pathways for psychic inhibition remain a mystery.

SITE B

An association between vascular lesions or tumors in the anterior temporal lobe of the brain and partial or total impotence with normal libido has recently been suggested.[25] Further clinical observations are needed to clarify the role of the anterior temporal lobe and other regions of the brain in the control of sexual functions.

SITE C

The relationship between spinal cord injury and erectile ability has already been discussed in detail. In complete cord lesions the ability to have either psychogenic or reflexogenic erections is selectively abolished, depending on whether there is a complete upper motor neuron lesion or a complete lower motor lesion of the sacral spinal cord, respectively. Theoretically, for spinal cord trauma to cause complete impotence, either both the thoracolumbar and sacral erection centers must be compromised or the psychic sequels to the trauma must be inhibiting the intact erection center.

SITE D

Multiple sclerosis commonly causes erectile dysfunction and even complete impotence. The latter implies rather widespread spinal cord damage, involving both erection centers (in the absence of psychic inhibition). Vas[42] showed that totally impotent men with multiple sclerosis may sweat in the upper extremities but do not sweat below the iliac crests, despite the presence of normal sweat glands in nonperspiring areas. This implies a disturbance of the autonomic outflow from the thoracolumbar cord, a disorder that apparently also frequently involves the penile erection centers that lie nearby.

SITE E

Tabes dorsalis is the form of neurosyphilis in which there is degeneration of the posterior (sensory) spinal roots, especially in the lumbosacral cord. From the physiological concepts presented earlier, these lesions should interfere with reflexogenic erections but not necessarily with psychogenic erections. Consequently, complete impotence is a relatively uncommon symptom of tabes dorsalis.[43]

SITE F

The incidence of erectile dysfunction in diabetes mellitus exceeds that in diabetic retinopathy or nephropathy.[44] In a random study of 200 diabetic men, 59 per cent were impotent.[45] The incidence of impotence does not correlate with the duration of the diabetes, the severity of the imbalance in carbohydrate metabolism, or the degree of diabetic control. Impotence is occasionally the initial clinical manifestation of diabetes,[46] and diabetes should be considered as a possible cause whenever a man complains of impotence. Ellenberg[45] found a high correlation between neurogenic bladder abnormalities and impotence and thereby postulated that an autonomic neuropathy was the cause of impotence in diabetes mellitus. Other causes of autonomic neuropathies are also frequently associated with impotence. Simpson[47] speculated that a diabetic angiopathy involving the small vessels of the erectile tissues might impede the blood flow and lead to impotence in some cases.

SITE G

Radical surgical procedures, such as abdominoperineal extirpation of the rectum, frequently destroy the nerve plexuses from both spinal erection centers, resulting in complete impotence. The effects of sympathectomy on potency, if any, have been discussed earlier. Other surgical procedures, such as transurethral prostate resection, that do not interfere with the neural or vascular structures mediating erection usually do not alter penile potency.[48,49]

SITE H

Drugs that inhibit the action of acetylcholine on structures innervated by postganglionic autonomic nerves (for example, methantheline bromide) occasionally cause impotence.[50] This effect is consistent with the role that cholinergic fibers play in opening the polsters and initiating erection.

SITE I

The association between thrombotic occlusion of the terminal aorta and impotence (components of Leriche's syndrome) is well known. Recently, impotence due to pelvic insufficiency alone has also been recognized.[51] The impotence in these cases is probably caused by an inability to maintain adequate rates of blood flow to the erectile tissues of the penis.

SITE J

Not only must there be an adequate arterial blood supply to the penis for erection to occur, but the erectile tissues must be capable of expanding to accommodate the increased blood flow. The thrombosed, fibrotic erectile tissues that are often the result of a prolonged priapism are not able to handle the increased blood flow. Therefore priapism may lead to complete impotence, although the ability to ejaculate remains intact.[52]

Many endocrine disorders, including hypopituitarism, eunuchoidism, myxedema, thyrotoxicosis, castration, Addison's disease, acromegaly, and adrenal feminization, have been associated with impotence. An alteration of libido frequently accompanies these disorders, and no doubt many of these cases of impotence are manifestations of psychic inhibition. For example, impotence does not necessarily follow bilateral orchiectomy; many patients who have been castrated as treatment for prostatic carcinoma have normal erections.[53] In lower mammals gonadal androgen influences the pre- and early post-natal organization of the neural tissue that mediates sexual behavior and sexual reflexes in the mature animal.[54] But penile erection occurs in infant monkeys and humans and can therefore be mediated by an immature central nervous system functioning under very low androgen levels.[55] It is evident that the development of higher cerebral function has progressively emancipated sexual function from strict gonadal control.[56] Thus the mechanism by which endocrine disorders as such produce impotence in man is unclear.

REFERENCES

1. Masters, W.H. and Johnson, V.E. Human Sexual Inadequacy. Boston, Little, Brown and Co., 1970, pp. 137-192.
2. Bors, F. and Comarr, A.F. Neurological disturbances of sexual function with special reference to 529 patients with spinal cord injury. Urol Survey 10:191-222, 1960.
3. Jovanovic U.J. The periodicity of erection during sleep in healthy men. Electroenceph Clin Neurophysiol 27:626, 1969.
4. Eckhardt, C. Untersuchungen über die Erection des Penis heim Hunde. Beitr Anat Physiol 3:123, 1863.

5. Kuntz, A. The Autonomic Nervous System, 4th ed. Philadelphia, Lea & Febiger, 1953, pp. 295-296.
6. Semans, J.H. and Langworthy, O.R. Observations on the neurophysiology of sexual function in the male cat. J Urol 40:836-846, 1938.
7. Pick, J. The Autonomic Nervous System. Philadelphia, J.B. Lippincott Co., 1970, p. 335.
8. Bors, E. and Comarr, A.E. Neurological Urology. Baltimore, University Park Press, 1971, p. 139.
9. Root, W.S. and Bard, P. The meditation of feline erection through sympathetic pathways with some remarks on sexual behavior after deafferentation of the genitalia. Am J Physiol 151:80-90, 1947.
10. Kuhn, R.A. Functional capacity of the isolated human spinal cord. Brain 73:1-51, 1950.
11. Zeitlin, A.B., Cottrell, T.L. and Lloyd, F.A. Sexology of the paraplegic male. Fertil Steril 8:337-344, 1957.
12. Munro, D., Horne, H.W. Jr. and Paull, D.P. The effect of injury to the spinal cord and cauda equina on the sexual potency of men. N Engl J Med 239:903-911, 1948.
13. Talbot, H.S. The sexual function in paraplegia. J Urol 73:91-100, 1955.
14. Bors, E. and Comarr, A.E. Effect of pudendal nerve operations on the neurologic bladder. J Urol 72:666-670, 1954.
15. Rose, S.S. An investigation in sterility after lumbar ganglionectomy. Br Med J 1:247-250, 1953.
16. Whitelaw, G.P. and Smithwick, R.H. Some secondary effects of sympathectomy: with particular reference to disturbance of sexual function. N Engl J Med 245:121-130, 1951.
17. Bacq, Z.M. Recherches sur la physiologie et la pharmacologie du système nerveux autonome. XII. Nature cholinergique et adrenérgique des diverses innervations vasomotrices du pénis chez le chien. Arch Int Physiol Biochem 41:311-321, 1935.
18. Dua, S. and MacLean, P.D. Localization for penile erection in medial frontal lobe. Am J Physiol 207:1425-1434, 1964.
19. MacLean, P.D. and Ploog, D.W. Cerebral representation of penile erection. J Neurophysiol 25:29-55, 1962.
20. MacLean, P.D., Denniston, R.H. and Dua, S. Further studies on cerebral representation of penile erection: caudal thalamus, midbrain, and pons. J Neurophysiol 26:273-293, 1963.
21. Robinson, B.W. and Mishkin, M. Penile erection evoked from forebrain structures in Macaca mulatta. Arch Neurol 19:184-198, 1968.
22. MacLean, P.D. Studies on the cerebral representation of certain basic sexual functions, in Brain and Behavior, vol. 3, edited by Gorski, R.A. and Whelan, R.E. Los Angeles, University of California Press, 1966, pp. 35-79.
23. Meyers, R. Three cases of myoclonus alleviated by bilateral ansotomy, with a note on postoperative alibido and impotence. J Neurosurg 19:71-81, 1962.
24. Tulane Department of Psychiatry and Neurology. Studies in Schizophrenia, Multidisciplinary Approach to Mind-Brain Relationships. Cambridge, Mass. Harvard University Press, 1954, pp. 235-251.

25. Hierons, R. and Saunders, M. Impotence in patients with temporal-lobe lesions. Lancet 2:761-763, 1966.
26. Terzian, H. and Ore, G.D. Syndrome of Klüver and Bucy reproduced in man by bilateral removal of the temporal lobes. Neurology 5:373-380, 1955.
27. Klüver, H. and Bucy, P.C. Preliminary analysis of functions of the temporal lobes in monkeys. Arch Neurol Psychiat 42:979-1000, 1939.
28. Alvarez-Morujo, A. Terminal arteries of the penis. Acta Anat (Basel) 67:387-398, 1967.
29. Henderson, V.E. and Roepke, M.H. On the mechanism of erection. Am J Physiol 106:441-448, 1933.
30. Conti, G. L'erection du penis human et ses bases morphologicovasculaires. Acta Anat (Basel) 14:217-262, 1952.
31. Newman, H.F., Northrup, J.D. and Devlin, J. Mechanism of human penile erection. Invest Urol 1:350-353, 1964.
32. Hotchkiss, R.S. and Fernandez-Leal, J. The nervous system as related to fertility and sterility J Urol 78:173-178, 1957.
33. Garrett, R.A. and Rhamy, D.E. Priapism: management with a corpus-saphenous shunt. J Urol 95:65-67, 1966.
34. O'Conor, V.J. Jr. Impotence and the Leriche syndrome: an early diagnostic sign; consideration of mechanism; relief by endarterectomy. J Urol 80:195, 1958.
35. Lowsley, O.S. and Bray, J.L. The surgical relief of impotence. JAMA 107:2029-2035, 1936.
36. Hart, B.L. and Kitchell, R.L. Penile erection and contraction of penile muscles in the spinal and intact dog. Am J Physiol 210:257-262, 1966.
37. Dorr, L.D. and Brody, M.J. Hemodynamic mechanisms of erection in the canine penis. Am J Physiol 213:1526-1531, 1967.
38. Bloom, W. and Fawcett, D.W. A Textbook of Histology, 9th ed. Philadelphia, W.B. Saunders Co., 1968, pp. 720-724.
39. Potts, J.F. The mechanism of ejaculation. Med J Aust 1:495-497, 1957.
40. Pond, H.S. Priapism as the presenting complaint of myelogenous leukemia: case report and review of the physiology of erection and the pathophysiology and treatment of priapism. Southern Med J 62:465-467, 1969.
41. Boerema, W.J. Priapism: case report and review of mechanism. Med J Aust 2:340-341, 1964.
42. Vas C.J. Sexual impotence and some autonomic disturbances in men with multiple sclerosis. Acta Neurol Scand 45:166-182, 1969.
43. Merritt, H.H., Adams, R.D. and Solomon, H.C. Neurosyphilis. New York, Oxford University Press, 1946, p. 246.
44. Koncz, L. and Balodimos, M.C. Impotence in diabetes mellitus. Med Times 98:159-170, 1970.
45. Ellenberg, M. Impotence in diabetes: the neurologic factor. Ann Intern Med 75:213-219, 1971.
46. Rubin, A. and Babbott, D. Impotence and diabetes mellitus. JAMA 168:498-500, 1958.
47. Simpson, S.L. Impotence. Br Med J 1:692-697, 1950.

24

48. Finkle, A.L. and Prian, D.V. Sexual potency in elderly men before and after prostatectomy. JAMA 196:139-143, 1966.
49. Gold, F.M. and Hotchkiss, F.S. Sexual potency following simple prostatectomy. New York J Med 69:2987-2989, 1969.
50. Schwartz, N.H. and Robinson, B.D. Impotence due to methantheline bromide. New York J Med 52:1530, 1952.
51. Canning, J.R., Bowers, L.M., Lloyd, F.A., et al. Genital vascular insufficiency and impotence. Surg Forum 14:298-299, 1963.
52. Money, J. and Hirsch, S. After priapism: organism retained, erection lost. J Urol 94:152-157, 1965.
53. Roen, P.R. Impotence: a concise review. New York J Med 65:2576-2582, 1965.
54. Hart, B.L. Neonatal castration: influence on neural organization of sexual reflexes in male rats. Science 160:1135-1136, 1968.
55. Beach, F.A. Cerebral and hormonal control of reflexive mechanisms involved in copulatory behavior. Physiol Rev 47:289-316, 1967.
56. Johnson, J. Impotence. Hospital Med 1:661-664, 1968.

3

Organic Impotence

ROGER T. CRENSHAW, M.D., DAVID E. MARTIN, PH.D.

HAROLD WARNER, AND THERESA L. CRENSHAW, M.D.

Impotence is the inability to obtain and sustain a penile erection. Unfortunately, some authors have added additional caveats to this simple definitional crux which are unnecessary and complicating. [15,28] Thus, it should not matter whether a male elicits the erection for masturbatory activities including ejaculation, or for heterosexual activities including coitus, or for homosexual activities. If he cannot erect his penis and maintain it erect for his purposes, then he is impotent.

Individuals with impotency can be grouped into two categories: organic (physiologic), where there is no accompanying psychologic problem, and psychogenic, where the reverse is true. Separation of cases has been made simpler by the studies of Karacan et al.[16] who showed by means of penile strain gauges that physiologically normal males have reflexogenic erections during sleep, especially REM sleep. If an individual can obtain such sleep-oriented erections, but cannot volitionally induce and maintain an erection upon trial, he is considered psychogenically impotent. There is nothing organically at fault with those anatomic and physiologic reflex processes which should allow him to obtain an erection. Similarly, if he does not obtain such sleep-oriented erections, and in addition cannot volitionally induce an erection, then he

The work described was partially supported by Grant No. MH28288 to the Yerkes Regional Primate Research Center of Emory University and to the Crenshaw Clinic by the National Institute of Mental Health.

is considered organically impotent. It is presumed, and usually discovered, that a specific disease process has prevented the normal erection mechanism from operating.

Components of both psychogenic and organic impotence may occur in a given individual, and this makes diagnosis and treatment not always an easy task. The male who becomes physiologically impotent will often develop significant psychological distress. Treating the primary cause alone will not necessarily be enough to reverse the impotence. However, it is essential to identify the organic component if it exists, because psychotherapy will not be effective in these cases. Even healthy individuals can have temporary periods of organic impotence arising from such factors as fatigue, alcohol ingestion, and incompatible environment.[12] In addition, there is a small incidence of iatrogenic organic impotency produced as an unwanted side effect of therapeutic drug administration[23] (anti-hypertensive drugs), specific surgery for non-related problems[1] (prostatic cancer), and therapy for non-related problems[21] (renal dialysis).

Organic impotence can be better understood by examining the mechanisms by which the various afflicting pathologies compromise the normal means by which erection is achieved. This chapter summarizes 1) the basic anatomic facts and physiologic processes concerning the genesis of erection (and ejaculation as well, in view of the functionally close relationship between the two); 2) the various reasons why organic impotence can occur when the physiologic processes are disrupted; and 3) the problems and possibilities for treatment of organic impotence. It will be evident that many organic diseases which result in impotence are not well understood in terms of how the disease—which may on the surface appear unrelated to the reproductive system—causes specific pathology to that system.

PHYSIOLOGY OF ERECTION AND EJACULATION

The mechanisms by which erection and ejaculation occur are complex, and in spite of both animal experimentation and clinical studies, the story has not completely unfolded. Some facts are clear. Erection is both a neuromuscular and a cardiovascular phenomenon, while ejaculation is solely neuromuscular.[9,10,30] Both can occur in spinal man, hence they are fundamentally reflex processes—involving spinal cord levels from T-12 to S-4. Superimposed upon this reflex level of activity, however, is a very important higher nervous system control, involving at least the cerebral cortex and very likely several other subcortical structures. Activity of these structures can either enhance or inhibit the activity of the reflex centers.

Reflex erection begins with stimulation of the glans penis, prostate, or urethra. Activation of a spinal reflex arc then occurs. The afferent limb involves the stimulated neurons, which are part of the pelvic and pudendal nerves, and synapse occurs in the sacral spinal cord. Here, in segments 2 to 4, efferent parasympathetic neurons are stimulated; these are often termed the *nervi erigentes*. They send impulses via the pelvic nerves and hypogastric plexus to the arteries responsible for circulation in the corpora cavernosa and spongiosa. The resulting arterial dilation increases circulation to these structures, and simultaneous venous compression impedes drainage. Hence tumescence occurs. Subsequent decrease in parasympathetic stimulation reinstates the normal arterial vessel caliber, because the vasoconstriction not only decreases arterial inflow but also enhances venous drainage of the corpora.

Ejaculation is an equally complex process, but solely neuromuscular.[9,10] It is best thought of as three separate but closely integrated mechanisms: 1) a peristaltic contraction of the smooth muscle lining the walls of the vasa deferentia as well as in the major sex accessory glands, i.e., prostate and seminal vesicles (release of semen by this type of contraction is often termed "emission"); 2) closure of the neck of the urinary bladder, again by smooth muscle contraction, to prevent retrograde movement of seminal fluid; and 3) clonic contractions of the bulbocavernosus and ischiocavernosus muscles which, if the preceding two mechanisms are functional, propels the seminal fluid rapidly through the urethra toward the exterior.

Both the sympathetic and parasympathetic portions of the autonomic nervous system are involved in accomplishing this triad of events, and two reflex arcs occur. One arc can be strictly peripheral, the afferent limb involving action potentials sent along the pudendal nerve to the spinal cord which activate efferent sympathetic neurons in the T-12 to L-3 regions. A central component of this arc can occur when the effects of pudendal nerve stimulation continue up the spinal cord to the cerebral cortex and back down to the T-12 to L-3 region. In normal man, both occur. Efferent sympathetic activation then courses to all involved structures—the vasa deferentia, prostate, seminal vesicles and bladder neck. Thus, emission and bladder neck closure should occur simultaneously, giving appropriate outward directional flow to the seminal fluid.

As this fluid moves into the prostatic and membranous portions of the urethra, receptor activation in the walls of this vessel, perhaps from the resultant distention or turgidity, initiates neural activity along the second reflex arc. Afferent fibers again are part of the pelvic and pudendal nerves, and synapse in the S-2 to S-4 region of the spinal cord. Synapse with somatic efferents innervating the bulbocavernosus and ischiocavernosus muscles causes their contraction clonically, and the seminal emission now becomes a propelled outflow.

Higher nervous system regulation and influence on erection and ejaculation is seldom mentioned in detail. This is not due to any lack of importance of higher neural inputs, but rather to a lack of precise data on the structures and mechanisms involved. It has been suggested that the cerebral cortex, hypothalamus, septum, and reticular formation are involved,[9,10] but further work is required to explain their specific interaction with the reflex centers.

With spinal cord transection, the reflex mechanisms can function independently of the higher brain centers, assuming there is adequate neural stimulation. When the spinal cord is intact, abnormal function of the higher centers can have inhibitory effects upon erection and ejaculation. Psychogenic impotency is a failure to achieve erection due to high level inhibition of the basic reflex mechanisms.

IMPOTENCY IN SPINAL CORD-INJURED PATIENTS

Injury to the spinal cord can result in serious neurophysiologic loss of both somatic and automatic function. The specificity of this loss is determined by the level of cord injury, and whether this injury has resulted in complete or incomplete lesions. The defects can be wide-ranging:[31] Horner's syndrome, cardiac symptoms, postural hypotension, gastrointestinal disturbance and others, but important among all of these is impairment of sexual function. Interference with erection can lead to impotence, while loss of ejaculation or testicular integrity can result in infertility.

Ample evidence in the literature attests to problems with erection and ejaculation in spinal cord-injured patients, as summarized in these important studies involving large patient populations:

Munro et al.[24] reported 84 male patients with traumatic lesions of the spinal cord; 74 per cent could still have erections, but only 7 per cent could ejaculate. Sacral lesions alone prevented erections, but ejaculation was often prevented when damage occurred at the T6-L3 cord level.

Talbot[26] studied 408 paraplegics during the late 1940's and early 1950's. More than two-thirds could achieve erection, one-third could achieve it in response to psychic stimuli; 15 per cent were infertile, due principally to ejaculatory inabilities. Sexual function disturbance, logically, was greater in those patients with injuries in the lumbosacral sexual reflex centers.

Zeitlin et al.[32] recorded 100 spinal cord-injured patients: 64

per cent could achieve complete erection, but only 3 per cent could ejaculate. Of the latter patients, none had lower thoracolumbar involvement.

Bors and Comarr[2] divided 529 patients into four groups according to the level and severity of the injury; upper motorneuron (UMN) lesions did not inhibit erection as much as did lower motorneuron (LMN) lesions. The mechanism by which erections were induced could be determined on the basis of whether there was a complete UMN lesion with sacral segments intact or a complete LMN lesion in the sacral segments or whether there was an incomplete lesion. Ejaculation was infrequent—19 per cent in LMN patients but only 8 per cent in UMN lesion subjects. They suggested that the sacral centers inhibit the activity of the thoracolumbar region, so that loss of higher facilitatory input due to an UMN lesion results in functional inhibition of the ejaculation process.

Thus, impotence and infertility both need to be reckoned with in sexual rehabilitation of the spinal cord-injured patient. This is especially true when one realizes that only one-third of cord-injured patients capable of inducing erections can maintain these sufficiently to accomplish coitus.[10] Methods need to be devised to adequately treat this aspect of impotence. Electrostimulation of the genital region via a rectal probe, as employed with lower animals for semen collection, stimulates both neural and muscular aspects of the prostate, seminal vesicles, vasa deferentia, urethra, and associated vascular system, as well as the skeletal muscles involved in penile erection (bulbocavernosus and ischiocavernosus), and if employed should be able to elicit both erection and ejaculation. However, technology regarding safe and intelligent use of electrical current for eliciting these phenomena in humans until now has not been available. We will shortly describe our ongoing research in this area.

ORGANIC IMPOTENCE IN PATIENTS OTHER THAN SPINAL CORD-INJURED

Impotence can arise secondary to many states of ill health, none of which initially involves the neuromuscular structures mediating erection. Masters and Johnson[22] established nine broad categories: anatomic (congenital deformities), cardiorespiratory (angina pectoris, emphysema, congenital and acquired heart disease), drug ingestion (tranquilizers, alpha-adrenergic blocking agents), endocrine (obesity, diabetes, thyrotoxicosis), genitourinary (prostatitis, carcinoma), hematologic (anemia, Hodgkin's disease), infectious (gonorrhea, mumps), neurologic (sympathectomy, parkinsonism, cord tumors), and vascular (arteritis, arteriosclerosis, embolus). Quite often, the report of impotence occurring with a particular disease entity involves only a few or even single case studies, and should be viewed at best as only a probability pending further documentation. Nevertheless, there are several important causes of secondary organic impotence[19] prevalent in the American population which deserve discussion.

Diabetes Mellitus. The incidence of impotence in diabetes has been variously estimated as 25 to 49 per cent,[19] and it apparently makes little difference whether the disease has an earlier or later onset. In a study of 175 male diabetics in an outpatient setting, Kolodny et al.[18] found that:

1. 49% were impotent; mean age was 50; duration of impotence was six years.
2. 2% had premature ejaculation.
3. 3% had retrograde ejaculation.
4. The onset of impotence was gradual over a period of six months to a year; however, interest in sexual activity was sustained.

There was no correlation between diet, duration of diabetes, type of hypoglycemic agent or diabetic control. This study supports Ellenberg's reports[8,9] which concluded that a neurologic basis for impotence existed in men with diabetes mellitus. In Ellenberg's study[8] of 45 diabetic impotent males with an average age of 43.2 years, 37 men had neurogenic bladder abnormalities and 38 men had demonstrable evidence of neuropathy. A random survey of 200 diabetic men showed 59 per cent to be impotent, and 82 per cent of these had neuropathy. These findings were also unrelated to the duration or severity of the diabetes. Plasma testosterone levels in both Ellenberg's and Kolodny's studies were normal, thus minimizing the probability of pituitary-gonadal axis failure as a plausible explanation.

The specific mechanism by which diabetes initiates peripheral neuropathy has been an enigma for many years, and is far from being reconciled. Two possibilities have been suggested: an obliteration of the blood vessels around neurons (vasa vasorum) and a metabolic problem in the Schwann cells.

The microvascular alterations which seem to occur almost everywhere suggest that an inability for proper engorgement of the penile cavernous sinuses might be due to vascular pathology.[7] However, other studies indicate that the relationship between the neuropathy and microangiopathy in diabetics is at best equivocal,[25] suggesting a metabolic alternative.

It is well known that Schwann cells are crucial for the maintenance of peripheral neuron integrity. The disruption of lipid metabolism by these cells due to insulin lack certainly supports their role in the neuropathy. But Greenbaum's report[13] of axonal degeneration as well as demyelination puts the idea of solely a segmental demyelination in doubt as well. Only by considerably more research and clinical study will this confused picture of the etiology of diabetic organic impotence be resolved.

Alcoholism. It is estimated that approximately nine million men and women are chronic alcoholics in the United States.[4] The acute effects of alcohol on the pituitary-gonadal axis have been defined[27] but the chronic effects of alcohol on sexuality are poorly understood. Lemere and Smith[20] studied 17,000 patients during a 37-year period and noted that of alcoholic men who were impotent, 50 per cent remained impotent following cessation of drinking, thus postulating the destructive effects of longterm alcoholism on the "reflex arc subserving erection." The mechanism by which chronic alcoholism leads to organic impotence is unknown.[23] In many patients suffering alcohol-induced hepatic cirrhosis, an endocrinologic basis for sexual dysfunction may exist due to estrogen-androgen imbalance.

Cardiovascular Disease and Hypertension. Many patients with cardiovascular disease receive pharmacologic agents to allay fears and anxieties, to improve cardiac status, to reduce high blood pressure or to combat side effects of arteriosclerotic vascular disease, such as intermittent claudication. Many of these drugs have been clearly implicated in impotence, retardation of ejaculation or retrograde ejaculation.[6,11,23]

Bulpitt and Dollery[3] reported that 67 per cent of patients taking bethanedine and 54 per cent taking guanethidine in an outpatient setting involving 477 hypertensive patients suffered impotence. Furthermore, failure of ejaculation occurred in 40 per cent of patients using bethanedine and in 58 per cent of those taking guanethidine.[3] Other studies support these conclusions.[17,19,23] The mechanism of this phenomenon may involve the unique degenerative response of the short adrenergic neurons found in the male reproductive tract when treated with alpha adrenergic blocking agents. A variety of agents appear to behave similarly, including in addition to guanethidine and bethanedine, reserpine and bretylium tosylate.

The AMA Committee on Hypertension[6] recorded data showing that patient non-compliance with prescribed therapeutic regimens is usually due to drug side effects. More current effort needs to be directed toward development of new drugs, or combinations of drugs, which minimize these side effects, including secondary organic impotence. One report[14] suggests, for example, that a combination of propranolol, hydralazine, and an oral diuretic is not only effective for controlling many cases of hypertension, but also has little associated incidence of impotence.

Renal Disease. Sexual adjustment to hemodialysis and renal transplantation has recently been delineated by Levy.[21] Of 778 patients who responded to a questionnaire, 59 per cent of male hemodialysis patients were impotent and 43 per cent of renal transplant patients were impotent. Most forms of acute renal disease are accompanied by feelings of lethargy and fatigue that decrease sexual activity, but the explanation for the impotence is not understood.

Treatment of Organic Impotence

Whereas psychogenic impotence can often be treated with remarkable success and speed through effective sexual psychiatric counseling, organic impotence poses more insurmountable problems. For many patients, their surgery (such as for prostatic carcinoma), the debilitation caused by their accompanying disease (e.g., diabetes, or the need for renal dialysis) makes the prognosis for cure of organic impotence low indeed. For some patients, medications which have less serious side effects in terms of impotence can often bring marked improvement.

The usual effective modality for treatment of physiologic impotence due to irreversible causes has been a surgical approach using medical silicone implants. This surgical technique has been improved greatly over the past five years, and an inflatable prosthesis developed by Scott and colleagues in Houston is a recent answer to many of the complaints about permanently rigid penile prosthetic devices.

Prosthetic devices are usually implanted in the corpora cavernosa bilaterally and extend into the crux posteriorly. Their splinting action on the penis allows for insertion into the vagina if desired, and ejaculation (if the male is physiologically capable of ejaculation). Surgical morbidity varies from a low of 5 per cent to a high of 25 per cent. Many patients require removal due to intolerance or infection; some patients need multiple procedures to effect permanent reversal of their impotence. However, the prosthetic implant is at this time the method of choice for reversal of organic impotence in selected patients.

RECENT RESEARCH IN RECTAL PROBE ELECTROSTIMULATION

Electrical stimulation through the rectum to activate reflex pathways involved in eliciting erection has been considered by many, but performed by only a few, with notably unsuccessful results. There has to date been no published study involving rectal probe electrostimulation of the human male which has recorded genesis of erection. The few existing reports of such attempts at electrical stimulus have not provided adequate information regarding current, voltage and tissue/electrode interface resistance even to permit useful analysis or repetition of the experiments. Following a highly successful study involving the use of rectal probe electrostimulation to elicit both erection and ejaculation in the great apes,[29] we began a study to adapt this procedure to the conscious human male. Initial studies with both healthy normal volunteers and volunteers with diseases or injuries involving impotence and problems with ejaculation have met with considerable initial success. Original data concerning results will appear in the scientific literature, but some preliminary details can be mentioned here.

The diameter of the rectal probe was 19mm, essentially the same as a sigmoidoscope. Two platinum electrodes were positioned longitudinally along the probe, their centers 120° apart. This allowed directional application of electric current into the tissue regions of interest, especially anterior structures such as the accessory sex glands and peripheral nerve pathways. Painful anal sphincter spasm during genital tissue stimulation was prevented by reducing to 4½mm the diameter of the probe in this sphincter region.

A sine wave generator in the frequency range of 0.1 Hz to 100 Hz supplied input to a 60-watt direct-current amplifier through a potentiometer which controlled the input intensity. The amplifier output was applied to the rectal probe electrodes through an electrical current-limiting device which positively opened the circuit when the delivered current rose above a predetermined maximum value. This prevented the possibility of accidental tissue damage.

Shock hazard was considered carefully in this study. Isolation transformers with electrostatic shields were employed wherever necessary. A special transformer exhibiting 140 decibels of common mode rejection of power-line transients (even lightning!) isolated the entire stimulating system from the building electrical mains.

Measurement of relevant electrical stimulus parameters permitted 1) precise knowledge of what was required to elicit erection, 2) comparison among individual subjects in order to examine norms and variations, and 3) duplication on different occasions by us and it is hoped by others interested in producing erection by this means. Highly accurate digital meters were employed to measure voltage and current, thereby allowing calculation of the electrode/tissue interface impedance. In order to measure alternating current at frequencies as low as 0.25 Hz, we developed a special meter which updated the root mean square value of the current at each half-cycle.

Results in both normal healthy males and paraplegic males with lesions at T-6 and below have indicated that erections can be induced via rectal probe electrostimulation, without invoking pain. Further work should serve to develop this tool to assist in the diagnosis of organic and psychogenic impotence, to assist organically impotent patients in obtaining erections, and even to elicit ejaculation in those desiring it.

REFERENCES

1. Belt, B.G. Some organic causes of impotence. Med. Aspects Hum. Sexuality 7:152, 1973.
2. Bors, E. and Comarr, A.E. Neurological disturbances of sexual function with special reference to 529 patients with spinal cord injury. Urol. Surv. 10:191, 1960.
3. Bulpitt, C.J. and Dollery, C.T. Side effects of hypotensive agents evaluated by a self-administered questionnaire. Br. Med. J. 3:485, 1973.
4. Calahan, D. and Cisin, I.H. American drinking practices: A national survey of behavior and attitudes related to alcoholic beverages. Rutgers Center of Alcohol Studies, Mongr. No. 6, New Brunswick, N.J.
5. Comarr, A.E. Sexual concepts in traumatic cord and cauda equina lesions. J. Urol. 106:375, 1971.
6. Committee on Hypertension of the American Medical Association: Drug treatment of ambulatory patients with hypertension. JAMA 225:1647, 1973.
7. Ditzel, J. Functional microangiopathy in diabetes mellitus. Diabetes 17:388, 1968.
8. Ellenberg, M. Impotence in diabetes: The neurologic factor. Ann. Intern. Med. 75:213, 1971.
9. Ellenberg, M. Impotence in diabetics: A neurologic rather than an endocrinologic problem. Med. Aspects Hum. Sexuality 7:12, 1973.
10. Fitzpatrick, W.F. Sexual function in the paraplegic patient. Arch. Phys. Med. Rehab. 55:221, 1974.
11. Freis, E.D. The chemotherapy of hypertension. JAMA 218:1009, 1971.
12. Goldberg, M. Selective impotence. Med. Aspects Hum. Sexuality 6:90, 1972.
13. Greenbaum, D. Observations on the homogenous nature and pathogenesis of diabetic neuropathy. Brain 87:201, 1964.
14. Howard, E.J. Sexual expenditures in patients with hypertensive disease. Med. Aspects Hum. Sexuality 7:82, 1973.
15. Johnson, J. Impotence. Br. J. Psychiat. Spec. Public. 9:206, 1975.
16. Karacan, I., Hursch, C.J. et al. Some characteristics of nocturnal penile tumescence in young adults. Arch. Gen. Psychiat. 26:351, 1972.
17. Kedia, K. and Markland, C. The effect of pharmacological agents on ejaculation, J. Urol. 114:569, 1975.
18. Kolodny, R.C., Kahn, C.B. et al. Sexual dysfunction in diabetic men. Diabetes 23:306, 1974.
19. Labby, D.H. Sexual concomitants of disease and illness. Postgrad. Med. 58:103, 1975.
20. Lemere, F. and Smith, J.W. Alcohol-induced sexual impotence. Am. J. Psychiat. 130:212, 1973.
21. Levy, N.B. Sexual adjustment to maintenance hemodialysis and renal transplantation. Trans. Am. Soc. Artif. Intern. Organs 19:138, 1973.
22. Masters, W.H. and Johnson, V.E. Human Sexual Inadequacy. Boston, Little, Brown, 1970, pp. 184-185.

23. Mills, L.C. Drug-induced impotence. Am. Family Physician 12:104, 1975.

24. Munro, D., Horne, H.W., Jr., and Paull, D.P. The effects of injury to the spinal cord and cauda equina on the sexual potency of men. N. Engl. J. Med. 239:903, 1948.

25. Pickering, G.W. The anatomical and functional aspects of the neurological lesions of diabetes. Proc. Roy. Soc. Med. 53:142, 1960.

26. Talbot, H.S. The sexual function in paraplegia. J. Urol. 73:91, 1955.

27. Toro, G., Kolodny, R.C. et al. Failure of alcohol to alter pituitary and target organ hormone levels. Clin. Res. 21:505, 1973.

28. Wabrek, A.J. and Wabrek, C.J. A primer on impotence. Med. Aspects Hum. Sexuality 10:102, 1976.

29. Warner, H., Martin, D.E. and Keeling, M.E. Electroejaculation of the great apes. Ann. Biomed. Eng. 2:419, 1974.

30. Weiss, H.D. Mechanism of erection. Med. Aspects Hum. Sexuality 7:28, 1973.

31. Whitelaw, G.P. and Smithwick, R.H. Some secondary effects of sympathectomy. N. Engl. J. Med. 245:121, 1951.

32. Zeitlin, A.B., Cottrell, T.L. and Lloyd, F.A. Sexology of paraplegic male. Fertil. Steril. 8:337, 1957.

4

The Handicapped and
Sexual Health

THEODORE M. COLE, M.D., SANDRA S. COLE, B.A.

Sexuality, like other birthrights, cannot be taken away by society. Society may channel sexual attitudes and expressions, but it cannot prohibit all the myriad forms and transformations generated by sexual energy. Society is now beginning to recognize that one's sexuality is not earned through work nor lost as an accident of injury or illness. Indeed, a news magazine recently reported that a radio station for the blind is broadcasting sexually explicit material to their audience who "are entitled to experience an array of literature they could respond to if they were not blind."[1]

The sexual birthright of everyone is the right to be curious, to experience and to learn about sex to the extent of one's initiative and ability to obtain information and cooperating partners while harming no one. Health professionals cannot really give back sexuality to their patients or clients. They can help people to understand their sexuality, to take responsibility for it and to make choices based on *information* and on *freedom from fear.*

ATTITUDES ABOUT DISABILITY AND SEXUALITY

What might cause a person to lose a sense of worthwhileness and the confidence and comfort that goes with it? Can physical disability have an adverse effect upon some aspects of the personality, such as sexuality? Can it influence sexual feelings such as comfort, competence, pleasure and desire? Or can the inverse be true? That is, can loss of a previous sexual identity create disability? We believe all are true. One feeds upon another and, if untreated, they act synergistically to deepen the problems of adjustment to the disability.

Although some physical disabilities directly affect sexuality by disablement of genital function, most do not.[2] Consider the effect of blindness upon sexual communication and fantasy. Imagine sexual partners, one of whom has recovered from a coronary, wanting freedom in sexual activities and fearing angina. Think about the young person with severe psoriasis, wanting acceptance and contact, but instead withdrawing and covering up his skin. Clearly, sexuality cannot be simply equated with genitality. In these examples sexuality is both defined by and expressed in how we present ourselves—our bodies, activities, relationships, preferences and aversions. Understood in these broad terms, it becomes clear that sexuality influences and is influenced by physical disability.

In the name of benevolence and protection, however, many people still take the position that sex information would "hurt" the disabled. Why should Pandora's box be opened to a person who is unable to use what is there? Isn't it better to avoid temptations and consequences? After all, disabled people are fragile and not expected to take care of themselves.

Certainly some disabilities produce physical and emotional vulnerabilities, but able-bodied and disabled people probably would not agree on a ranking of those vulnerabilities. The reasoning above is typical of protective parent role played by society to the detriment of the disabled and the able-bodied alike. Sex educators have long known that the wish to protect others from the dangers of sexual information is often an expression of the anxiety within the protector that is transferred to the target groups of young, mentally retarded, disabled, or elderly individuals whom society believes to be unable to take care of themselves!

In our efforts to protect, we sexually disenfranchise the people we are trying to benefit. Consider the adolescent with congenital brain injury who lies on the examining table in the doctor's office, where attention is directed towards physical restoration of the hand, the leg or speech, but seldom toward sexual development. Major treatment facilities for disabled children continue to overlook the sexuality of their clients and, when asked to do something, react in anger and dismay.

Yet to neglect the sexuality of the disabled adolescent is to give the cloaked message that sexuality is neither expected nor appropriate for that person.[3] With these threads of sexuality dropped, what holes do we leave in the fabric of maturation? Young individuals are asked to cope with their disabilities while being denied access to information about the adult world which flourishes around them, and which uses sexual communication as a frequent part of daily living.

RELATIONSHIP OF PHYSICAL DISABILITY TO SEXUALITY

Type of disability : **Progressive**
Time of onset : **Early life, Prepuberty**

	Masturbation	Coitus	Fertility	Conspicuous to Society
Diseases of the Brain			♂ ♀	♂ ♀
Diseases of the Spinal Cord	♂ ♀	♂	♂	♂ ♀
Musculo - Skeletal Diseases	♂ ♀	♂ ♀	♂	♂ ♀
Metabolic or Deficiency Diseases				♂ ♀
Heart Disease				♂ ♀
Blindness				♂ ♀
Deafness				♂ ♀

Symbols (♂♀) indicate for each sex the conspicuousness and the areas of sexual function which are often significantly affected by progressive physical disabilities with onset in early life.

How can disabled adolescents learn the social skills of our complex society if they are unable to utilize the community to obtain information and awareness as other young people do? How likely is it that the disabled will risk their own vulnerability by attempting to become part of a society which limits their coping tools? If handicapped people are kept out of sight, how can the able-bodied majority in our society ever learn that *these citizens are human beings who have a right to information and to full participation in our society?* People with one or more physical handicaps do not need another one imposed upon them by a society which, for the most part, is insensitive to the sexual needs of the disabled.

For some, however, disability offers an opportunity to better understand one's self.[4] Reassessment of one's own ingrained attitudes is not often undertaken by most adults. The average person may have little reason to reassess his sexuality since "it all seems to be working pretty well for me." Reason to do so usually arrives on the wings of crisis, disruption and pain. Only when the old rules are changed and the solutions of the past no longer apply do some begin to re-examine the foundations of their sexuality.

Imagine yourself with chronic renal failure and secondary impotence or with multiple sclerosis and incontinence. In that imaginary world one may find compelling reasons to re-examine the notions that a beautiful body or a stiff penis are essential to a satisfactory sex life. The exploring mind may perceive some of the richness of sexuality and sexual relationships which may have been hidden behind society's well known external symbols of maleness and femaleness, of desirability and acceptability.

Just how far this reconsideration of sexuality may carry a person is an individual matter, but in spite of the liabilities imposed by a handicapping condition, it may contain the potential for enrichment. Some disabled people report that they might have overlooked this potential for enrichment had they not become physically disabled.

IMPLICATIONS FOR HEALTH PROFESSIONALS

The implications of what is written here fall most heavily upon those in the health care system who set health care policies for the physically disabled, especially the chronically disabled. The authors are most familiar with the medical rehabilitation setting and will explore implications within that context. However, the implications are similar, if not identical, for other settings such as counseling, community work, administration and management, government, etc.

Some of the attitudes and practices of the helping professions merit consideration. *Health practitioners first must be comfortable with their*

own sexuality before they can be helpful to others with sexual con-
cerns. Consider the physician who, thinking it inappropriate, refuses to
discuss sex with his patients. Many doctors hope that someone else
with more skill will see the need and provide the service. If physicians
fail to recognize that most disabled people want the honest information
which will help them function in an able-bodied world, then the patient
may not find help. Would it not be wiser for the physician to initiate
discussion, provide information and affirm sexuality as a part of emotional health?

A nurse who believes that the sexuality of a patient is strictly a private matter will avoid the topic. What happens when professional helpers smother a patient's genuine questions about sex under a treatment
program that includes only physical therapy or vocational rehabilitation? In doing so, they overlook the fact that sex, as a natural part of
life, deserves encouragement and belongs in the client's treatment plan.

Attending to sexual awareness, function and responsibility can help
people learn, just as they learn from attending to other coping techniques. *If sexual comfort is taught, sexual competence may result.*
Many disabled people are in primary relationships when they come to
treatment centers and could benefit from an enlightened, supportive approach to the sexual aspects of their disability. Help may be provided
by a social worker who knows that the patient's probings about reproduction may also be questions about sexuality. Communication with a
disabled patient or client may be improved by a practitioner who displays a willingness to discuss his or her own sexuality.

Medical rehabilitation has been defined in many ways. In considering
sexuality and physical disability, we believe that it is a process which
promotes the stabilization of the disabling condition and assists in regaining those abilities which allow resumption of maximum responsibility for one's own life. If the disability is complex or moderately
severe, the fulfillment of this definition will require the efforts of an integrated team of practitioners who can provide an array of health care
services in medical, psychosocial, vocational and educational areas.
Such a team will discover that fruitful work with the chronically disabled mandates a rapport of trust and open communication which must
be maintained over the duration of the disability and its treatment.
Trust is not easily achieved and may be hampered by aloofness, impaired communication, or distance between the professional and the
client. Sensitive attention given to sexuality, however, can play a facilitating role in building rapport by emphasizing warmth and openness
and minimizing aloofness and barriers to communication. After all, if
we can talk about sex, we can talk about anything!

Sex can be a leveler—an equalizer—among people. It can help minimize the parent/child relationship which so often characterizes the attitudes between the health care team and the client. It is difficult, if not impossible, to regard a disabled person as dependent and childlike while simultaneously recognizing his or her sexual expectations and need for sexual skills. Helping clients to understand their own responsibility in finding sexual satisfaction may foster self-responsibility, maturity and positive actions toward other rehabilitation goals.

If one accepts that there is a relationship between sexuality and the adjustment of the disabled person to other aspects of life, then there is a clear need to prepare professionals to deal with sexuality, their own and their clients', and to integrate sexual health into the health care system. In this regard, the dominant need of health care professionals is to better understand their own sexuality in order to utilize their resources and awarenesses in the treatment of others.[6] There are a variety of educational programs in the United States which help the professional understand sexuality—his, hers and theirs.[7] Augmenting these programs is an expanding literature which can help one reassess sexual attitudes.

Practitioners who allow themselves the fantasy of their own physical disability, often develop a willingness to consider the sexuality of others. In fantasy one can have a colostomy, amputated leg, loss of sensation, painful deformity or life-threatening health concern. Try superimposing one of these disabilities onto your recent sexual activities. You can then begin to feel vicariously the significance of your body in an intimate relationship with another person whose approval is vital to your self-esteem.

After attitudes are re-examined and understood, information can be provided which equips the practitioner to deal with those aspects of sexuality which might be affected by physical disabilities. Specific counseling skills which may help to improve the sexual attitude and function of the disabled client can be learned. The education of the practitioner should also include the opportunity to practice these skills so that they will have the effect he wants.

All health practitioners who work with the physically disabled should have the attitudes, information and skills which provide permission for people to have a problem and to explore it. Other professionals will have the additional ability to provide limited services. And, some practitioners will learn the extensive skills needed to deal with the specific sexual problems that a physically disabled client may have. At all of these three levels—permission, limited services or extensive skills—the practitioner should know when to refer the patient to another colleague who has special skills.

SOME GUIDELINES FOR THE HANDICAPPED

There are some guidelines which may help the practitioners and the client in learning about the sexuality of physical disability.[8]

A stiff penis does not make a solid relationship, nor does a wet vagina.

Urinary incontinence does not mean genital incompetence.

Absence of sensation does not mean absence of feelings.

Inability to move does not mean inability to please.

The presence of deformities does not mean the absence of desire.

Inability to perform does not mean inability to enjoy.

Loss of genitals does not mean loss of sexuality.

Everyone has the right to be sexual. We encourage practitioners to include in their health care the information and competencies which can enable the disabled to take responsibility for their own lives, including their sexual lives. Sexual health cannot be separated from total health.

REFERENCES

1. Rockwell, M. "The Washington Air." Newsweek, October 27, 1975.
2. Cole, T.M. Sexuality and the Physically Handicapped in Human Sexuality: A Health Practitioner's Text. Green, R. (Ed.), Baltimore, Williams & Wilkins Co., 1975.
3. Blos, P. Jr. and Finch, S.M. Sexuality and the Handicapped Adolescent in The Child With Disabling Illness: Principles of Rehabilitation, Downey, J.A., Low, N.L. Philadelphia, W.B. Saunders Co., 1974.
4. Cole, T.M., Chilgren, R. and Rosenberg, P. A New Program of Sex Education and Counseling for Spinal Injured Adults and Health Care Professionals. Int. J. Para, Aug 1973. pp. 111-124.
5. Mooney, T., Cole, T.M. and Chilgren, R. Sexual Options for Paraplegics and Quadriplegics. Boston, Little, Brown & Company, 1975.
6. Cole, T.M. and Cole, S.S. Sexuality and Physical Disabilities: The Physician's Role. Minnesota Med. (In press)
7. Lief, H.I. Why Sex Education for Medical Students? in Human Sexuality: A Health Practitioner's Text, Green, R. (Ed.) Baltimore, Williams & Wilkins Co., 1975.
8. Anderson, T.P., Cole, T.M. and Chilgren, R. Sexual Counseling of the Physically Disabled. Post Grad. Med., July 1975, pp. 117-123.

5

Sexual Impotence and Some Autonomic Disturbances in Men with Multiple Sclerosis

C.J. VAS

Clinical neurologists have been aware for a long time that patients with multiple sclerosis (MS) often complain of sexual impotence. This complication is frequently encountered in severely disabled men who have had MS for many years. During the therapeutic trials conducted recently at Leeds, England, the incidence of impotence was found to be high even though the subjects were not severely incapacitated by MS. The frequency of impairment of sexual potency was therefore estimated in the patients admitted to the trials and various aspects of their autonomic and testicular functions were investigated. The findings are reported in the following study.

   Definitions. The definition of impotence conformed to the suggestion of *Masters & Johnson* (1966). These authors defined impotence as a disturbance of sexual function in the male that precluded satisfactory coitus. It varied from a total loss of erective prowess (total impotence*) to an inability to attain or maintain full erection (partial impotence*). Furthermore, impotence was classified as primary if it had been present from the onset of sexual activities or as secondary if the difficulty had followed a history of effective sexual function. At this stage, it must be

―――――――――――――

*The terms in parentheses are used throughout this chapter.

noted that all the sexually disabled patients included in this report complained of secondary impotence.

Selection of patients. The subjects selected had unequivocal clinical features of MS based on evidence of lesions disseminated in time and space over a span of years in the central nervous system. Corroborative evidence was often also obtained after examination of the cerebrospinal fluid. In an attempt to exclude severely disabled men, patients requiring the use of a walking stick or those unable to work or continue the normal activities of living were not investigated. In addition, all the subjects had to be capable of being up and about for at least 12 hours in the day (viz. Grade 5, Kurtzke 1961).

Clinical Data. The ages of the 37 patients studied ranged from 18 to 50 years with a mean of 39 years. All the men apparently had normal libidinous desires. The incidence of total or partial impotence is shown in Table 1 from which it will be seen that 43.2 per cent of the men complained of some degree of impotence.

Table 1. Variation in sexual potency of 37 male patients between the years 1965 and 1966.

	1965		1966
Totally impotent	3		2
		43.2%	
Partially impotent	13		15
Normally potent	21		20
Total	37		37

Variation between 1965-1966

Totally impotent	→ partially impotent:	1
Partially impotent	→ normality:	1
Normally potent	→ partially impotent:	2
Total		4

The average age and duration of MS in the normal and impotent groups of men are summarized in Table 2. The small numbers and inequality of patient-groups were felt to preclude a meaningful statistical analysis which was therefore not undertaken. Nevertheless, it will be obvious that the demyelinating process had been present for a longer period (12 years) in the totally impotent patients than the partially impotent (9 years) or the normally potent men (5.5 years).

Table 2. (Age range: 18-50 years)

	Average duration of Multiple Sclerosis (years)	Average age (years)
Totally impotent	12	40
Partially impotent	9	39.5
Normally potent	5.5	36.5

The abnormal neurological findings in all patients with MS were assessed according to the Kurtzke Disability Scale (*Kurtzke* 1961). The averages of the disabilities under the overall disability (K), pyramidal (P), cerebellar (Cll), brainstem (BS), sensory (S) and bowel-bladder functions (BoBl) are recorded in Table 3. From an inspection of this table, it appeared that there was a significant difference in the abnormalities of sensation and bowel-bladder function between the impotent men on the one hand and the partially impotent and normally potent men on the other. A more detailed analysis of the sensory abnormalities of the impotent individuals revealed that the difference in the findings was due to the greater involvement of the spinothalamic system. It was also observed that the totally impotent men complained more frequently of incontinence or retention of urine than either of the other two groups of patients. The partially impotent men were more liable to urgency or incontinence of urine than their sexually normal counterparts. It should be pointed out at this stage that urethral catheterization had not been attempted for the relief of urinary retention in any patient prior to the investigation of sexual function and a past history of orchitis could not be obtained in any subject, except one potent male who had previously developed orchitis in association with mumps.

Table 3. Average disability of patients on Kurtzke scale.

	K.	Pyr.	Cll.	BS.	S.	Bo.Bl.
Impotent	4	3	2	2	3	3
Partially impotent	3	3	2	1	1.5	1.5
Potent	3	3	2	1	1	<0.5

K. = Kurtzke overall disability. Pyr. = pyramidal. Cll. = cerebellar.
BS. = brain-stem. Bo.Bl. = bowel-bladder.

METHODS

Autonomic Function: During the examination of the autonomic nervous system in the 37 patients, particular emphasis was laid on the clinical presence of orthostatic hypotension and the state of sudomotor function.

A history of symptoms suggestive of postural hypotension was asked for in all the patients with MS. In addition, the blood pressure was estimated with a sphygmomanometer cuff on the arm and the subjects made to change position rapidly from the supine to the erect.

Sudomotor Function: Thirty-seven patients were investigated. Each subject was examined in a heated room. A cup of hot tea and oral aspirin (600 mg) were initially given to expedite a sweating response. Each patient was then instructed to lie supine on a bed when quinizarin powder (*Guttmann* 1947) was sprayed on the anterior aspect of the whole body including the perineum. Thereafter, an electric heating bed-cradle was placed above the subject. Both the cradle and the patient from the neck down were then covered with blankets. The onset and location of perspiration was demonstrated by the appearance of a blue color following the interaction of the sweat and the quinizarin powder. The heating was stopped if the patient perspired freely all over the front of the body or as soon as the skin developed an erythematous appearance in the non-perspiring areas. At that stage the quinizarin was wiped off, the patient made to lie prone, quinizarin re-sprayed on the back of the body and the heating recommenced and continued until the patient once again perspired freely or developed erythema.

Pilocarpine nitrate (7.5 mg) was administered intravenously (*List & Peet* 1938) after an adequate interval if thermoregulatory sweating did not appear on the face, neck, trunk, perineum or extremities. The appearance of the sweating was again noted by the alteration in color of the sprayed quinizarin. Subsequently, in 7 impotent patients, 0.1 ml of 1:1000 acetylcholine (*Bennett & Scott* 1965) was injected intradermally in the areas where thermoregulatory sweating was absent to determine the integrity of the post-ganglionic autonomic nerve fibers (*Rothman & Coon* 1939, *Coon & Rothman* 1940). Finally, heat was applied with a hot water bottle (*Janowitz & Grossman* 1950) and quinizarin sprayed on those areas of skin that did not perspire, despite all the previous procedures, in an attempt to demonstrate the presence or absence of sweat glands. These tests for sudomoter function were performed twice with an interval of 12 months between the years of 1965 and 1966. The results were correlated with the state of sexual potency. In recording the results, the term 'sweat loss' referred to totally absent or grossly deficient sweating in a given area.

Urinary gonadotrophins: Both follicle-stimulating and interstitial cell stimulating hormones were estimated in 31 patients by Dr. G.W. Pennington using 2 immature mice for each estimation (*Brown* 1955). As the normal range varies widely for the different ages of men (Table 4), only values in excess of 70 mouse-units were arbitrarily considered as abnormal.

Lumbo-sacral autonomic reflexes: The scrotal, bulbo-cavernosus and anal sphincter reflexes were examined in the 31 subjects with MS in whom the urinary gonadotrophins were assayed.

Table 4. Normal urinary gonadotrophin (U.G.) values for different ages in men.

Ages (years)	U.G. range (mouse-units)	Mean
14-25	3-38	7
25-44	3-38	15
44-54	5-50	17
55-64	6-67	21
65-74	8-75	29
75-96	5-70	18

RESULTS

Sudomotor Function: Three patterns of sweating were observed in the 37 male subjects. The 21 normally potent men were found to perspire freely all over the body. The 13 partially impotent men perspired on the face, neck, trunk and perineum but not on the lower extremities. The 3 impotent men however did not sweat between the iliac crests. There were two exceptions to these findings. The thermoregulatory sweating pattern of a partially impotent subject in 1965 was abnormal since he perspired on the face, neck, arms, chest and over the gross varicosities in his legs but not on his abdomen, perineum, thighs or feet. However, an intradermal injection of acetylcholine into the abdominal wall and thighs did result in local sweating, thus showing that the postganglionic nerves were intact. In addition, following the administration of pilocarpine, sweating appeared all over the body. One year later, his potency had returned to normal and the sweating pattern had reverted to that expected of a normally potent man. The second exception will be referred to when discussing the findings at the time of the re-examination 12 months later. Two totally impotent and 5 partially impotent men were subjected to intradermal injections of acetylcholine in those areas of skin which did not show thermoregulatory sweating. Following the procedure, sweating occurred around the site of the injection.

The presence of sweat glands in the non-perspiring areas was confirmed in all impotent and partially impotent subjects by the alteration in color of the quinizarin powder following the injection of pilocarpine intravenously. The absence of sweat glands in areas such as the lateral aspects of the thighs and legs was noted in 2 individuals by the absence of sweating after the application of local heat with a hot water bottle.

At the time of the re-examination of all subjects in 1966, a variation in potency of 4 patients was noted (Table 1). One male who was apparently totally impotent in 1965 had improved to a state of partial impotence. In this subject, the sweat-pattern had also changed from that seen in the study with totally impotent men to that encountered in partially impotent subjects. Another patient, normally potent in 1965, was stated to have become partially impotent but his sweat-pattern had not altered from the normal appearance observed in 1965. However, when examined neurologically, it was found that this man was analgesic from the costal margins down to the feet. A third normally potent man who perspired freely in 1965 had deteriorated and become partially impotent with the accompanying alteration of the sweat-pattern to that consistent with the partially impotent state in this study. The fourth individual on the other hand improved from being partially impotent to a normally potent state. His sweat-pattern also reflected the improvement as it changed from being abnormal in 1965 to a completely normal picture in 1966.

Table 5. Distribution of urinary gonadotrophin levels in 31 patients.

		Elevated gonadotrophins (>70 mouse units)	Normal gonadotrophins	Per cent
Impotent	(3)	2	1	66.6
Partially impotent	(11)	3	8	37.5
Normally potent	(17)	1 (physiological)	16	0
Total	(31)			

Autonomic: No history of postural hypotension was obtained in any patient, nor did orthostatic hypotension occur when the patients rapidly changed from a supine to an erect posture.

Urinary Gonadotrophins: The urinary gonadotrophin levels in 31 patients are summarized in Table 5. Approximately 66 per cent of the impotent and 37 per cent of the partially impotent patients had elevated urinary gonadotrophins. The normally potent subject with a previous history of "mumps-orchitis" resulting in sterility was also found to have abnormally elevated urinary gonadotrophins. On the other hand, the urinary gonadotrophins were not elevated in normally potent patients with MS.

Lumbo-sacral reflexes: The scrotal, bulbo-cavernosus and anal sphincter reflexes were examined in the 31 patients in whom the urinary gonadotrophins were also assayed. These reflexes, dependent on an intact lumbo-sacral system, were used to check the integrity of their respective neural pathways. The results are summarized in Tables 6, 7 and 8 for the three different groups of patients, *i.e.* impotent, partially impotent and normally potent men respectively. The scrotal, cremasteric and bulbo-cavernosus reflexes were absent in all 3 impotent men.

On the other hand, they were intact in the majority of normal men, although they were more frequently abnormal in the partially impotent subjects with elevated gonadotrophin levels in the urine.

Loss of ejaculatory power occurred in all of the totally impotent men and in about 30 per cent of the partially impotent subjects.

Table 6. Reflexes in impotent men (3 patients).
Gonadotrophin levels abnormally high in 2 patients:
at upper limit of normal in 1 patient (*).

	Absent	Present	Doubtful($\pm$)
Scrotal	3		
Bulbocavernosus	3		
Anal sphincter	1	1(*)	1

Table 7. Reflexes in partially impotent men (11 patients).
Abnormally high Gonadotrophin levels (3 patients).

	Absent	Present	Doubtful($\pm$)
Scrotal		3	
Bulbocavernosus	1		2
Anal sphincter	1		2

Normal Gonadotrophin levels (8 patients).

	Absent	Present	Doubtful($\pm$)
Scrotal	5	3	
Bulbocavernosus	6	1	1
Anal sphincter	7	1	

Table 8. Reflexes in normally potent men (17 patients).

	Present	Absent
Scrotal	15	2
Bulbocavernosus	17	—
Anal sphincter	17	—

DISCUSSION

There is little doubt that sexual impotence can occur as a result of the demyelinating lesions seen in MS. Ivers & Goldstein (1963) reported that impotence occurred in 26 per cent and was the presenting symptom in 3 per cent of all the patients with MS seen at the Mayo Clinic. Little detailed information is however available with respect to the incidence, site of the causative lesion, associated abnormalities and treatment, if any.

It must be emphasized that the adoption of strict diagnostic criteria resulted in only a small number of patients with an unequivocal diagnosis of MS being selected for investigation. Severely disabled patients, unable to walk without aid, were also excluded. This restriction was thought advisable in order to determine the incidence of neurogenic impotence in comparatively well preserved males with normal libido. For the same reason, patients who had either been catheterized previously, or those who had contracted orchitis secondary to an infection of the urinary tract, were not included.

The incidence of neurogenic impotence (partial and total) in this highly selected series of patients with normal libido and ages ranging from 18-50 years was 43.2 per cent. It is however not unlikely that the incidence of this symptom might have been greater if severely incapacitated patients had been surveyed. This finding of impotence in 43 per cent of patients is in marked contrast to the predictions of *Kinsey* and his associates (1948) who suggested that only 6.7 per cent of normal men up to the age of 54 years were impotent.

It has been the impression of some authorities that impotence usually develops late in the natural history of MS. Table 2 clearly shows that the totally impotent men had been victims of MS for a longer period (12 years) than either the partially impotent men who had the disease for 9 years or the normally potent men with MS of 5.5 years duration.

Impotence may remit (Table 1), as was seen to occur in one totally impotent and another partially impotent individual in this small series.

Investigation of thermoregulatory sweating in the sexually normal subjects showed that they perspired normally all over the body. The totally impotent men did not perspire below the waist, whereas the partially impotent individuals perspired on the face, upper limbs and trunk, including the perineum and groins but not on the lower limbs. The intradermal injection of acetylcholine in 7 patients with abnormal patterns of sweating and the intravenous administration of pilocarpine in all the sexually normal subjects demonstrated satisfactorily the integrity of the postganglionic nerves and the presence of effectively functioning sweat glands, respectively, in those areas of skin where sweating was not previously observed. Intradermal testing with acetylcholine was not attempted in all affected subjects because of the reluctance of patients to undergo a somewhat painful procedure. The implication of the acetylcholine test results may however be applicable to other patients with abnormalities of sweating.

Anhydrosis is due to a lesion located either in the central nervous system or peripherally in the sympathetic outflow. The plaques of demyelination seen in MS are characteristically found in the central nervous system and not in the peripheral nervous system or even in the sympathetic chain of ganglia (*Lumsden* 1966). It is therefore unlikely that the absence of sweating seen in patients with MS would have a dermatome arrangement as mapped out by *Head & Campbell* (1900), *Foerster* (1933) and *Richter & Woodruff* (1945). On the contrary, it is suggested that the abnormal patterns of sweating in MS would not be consistent with a "lower motor neurone" lesion of the sympathetic system but rather with that of an "upper motor neurone" type. There is however no reliable information with regard to the latter state. *Foerster* (1936) and *Guttman* (1931) observed anhydrosis after anterolateral chordotomy. *Johnson et al.* (1952) concluded from a small series of patients that abnormalities in sudomotor function without a dermatome pattern may occur as a result of lesions in the anterolateral quadrant of the spinal cord. *Gillilan* (1955) stated that lesions of the ventral reticulospinal tracts caused impairment or loss of sweating not necessarily having a dermatome pattern, due to an interference of function in either the ventral reticulospinal pathways or more likely in the fiber-tracts in the anterolateral columns of the cord and presumably their lateral horn connections.

Although a precise location of the lesions is not possible in the patients studied by the author, it may be assumed that the defect is in the central nervous system somewhere between the hypothalamic area and the thoracolumbar cord. The presence of sweating on the upper limbs and the upper part of the trunk does however imply that the abnormality probably involves the dorsolumbar cord itself or those central fibers which terminate in that area.

Penile erection and ejaculation of semen are sexual reflexes mediated by the autonomic nervous system. *Semans & Langworthy* (1938) observed from their experiments in cats that ejaculation consists of two distinct actions, the first being emission of semen into the urethra due to the sudden contraction of the smooth muscle of the internal genital organs. The second part of ejaculation is a term used in a mechanistic sense to describe the expulsion of semen from the urethra by contraction of the striped bulbo-cavernosus muscle. The reflex arc for ejaculation is mediated by afferent sense organs in the glans penis which send impulses to the upper part of the lumbar cord via the pudendal nerves. The efferent impulses from the upper lumbar segments are propagated through the lumbar communicating rami and the hypogastric nerves to the smooth and striped muscles involved in ejaculation. Ejaculation therefore cannot be elicited after destruction of the lumbar cord or by division of either the sympathetic nerves to the pelvic organs or the pudendal nerves.

Penile erection occurs whenever the cavernous bodies of the penis are engorged with blood. This reflex phenomenon can be initiated by either direct sensory stimulation of the glans or by psychic stimuli transmitted from the cerebral cortex. The sensory impulses may flow along the pudendal nerve to a lumbar center whereas the psychic stimuli from the cortex traverse the diencephalon and spinal cord to terminate in the same lumbar centre. At this stage, impulses may flow along the sympathetic outflow (S2-4) to the vascular supply of the penis producing dilatation of the vessels, engorgement of the sinuses and passive compression and retardation of the venous outflow. In addition, the lumbar center may produce an inhibition of the sympathetic vasoconstrictor fibers. However, erection can still occur after sympathetic denervation of the penis (*Kuntz* 1946).

It is well established from animal experimentation that a sacral center (parasympathetic) mediates erection and that a lumbar center (sympathetic) is responsible for ejaculation (*Kuntz* 1946). It must be noted in addition that reflex erection will not occur (*i.e.* impotence) in cats following stimulation of the glans if the pudendal nerve is divided (*Semans & Langworthy* 1938). Likewise, according to *Semans & Langworthy* (1938) and *Kuntz* (1946), psychic stimulation will produce erection despite the destruction of the sacral cord but not after the destruction of the lumbar cord. These findings were confirmed by *Root & Bard* (1947) in male cats deprived of the central sacral connections of the nervi erigentes. These animals developed full erections on seizing and attempting to mount oestrous females. The authors proposed that an intact suprasacral vasodilator outflow originating chiefly from the 2nd, 3rd and 4th lumbar cord segments was essential for erection to occur. It may therefore be assumed that an intact lumbar cord is essential for mediation of penile erection.

Erection may result from sensory impulses originating in the region of the glans penis or from psychic impulses arriving at an erection center (sacral-parasympathetic) after traversing an intact lumbar cord. In the case of the patients with MS, it is of interest that neither reflex sensory nor psychic erection occurred in the totally impotent. On the other hand, both sensory and psychic erection were reported but were not sustained enough for satisfactory intromission to occur in the partially impotent.

The findings of *Zeitlin* and his co-workers (1957) are germane to the present investigation. These authors examined 100 male paraplegic patients with complete cord lesions either in the cervical, dorsal or lumbar areas. It was found in this group that total and partial impotence occurred with the greatest frequency when the cord lesion was in the lumbar area, the lowest incidence being seen with cervical cord lesions. Unfortunately, *Zeitlin et al.* (1957) did not investigate the sudomotor function in their patients.

Bors and his co-workers (1950) examined in some detail 34 paraplegic subjects with complete (20 patients) and incomplete (14 patients) lesions in the cervical thoracic, lumbar and sacral areas. These authors were of the opinion that testicular atrophy corresponded well with abnormalities of sweating. They reported that lesser testicular pathology was associated with normal sweating and major testicular pathology with impaired sweating indicating a direct relationship between testicular function and the autonomic nervous system. However, they found no correlation between biopsy findings and sexual behaviour. The present work differs from that of Bors et al. (1950) who did not apparently attempt a specific correlation between abnormalities of sweating and penile erection.

It is suggested after a consideration of the pathophysiology of the sexual reflexes and the clinical reports on impotence referred to above, that the lesion producing impotence in patients with MS is in the spinal cord, either in the cervical, dorsal or lumbar areas.

Johnson and his co-workers in England (1966) described two patients with progressive and diffuse neurological diseases accompanied by orthostatic hypotension, impotence and loss of sweating. The abnormal pattern of sweating was not ascertained. At post-mortem examination a significant degree of nerve-cell loss in the intermediolateral columns (preganglionic sympathetic cells) of the dorsolumbar cord was observed. The absence of postural hypotension in the subjects with MS may be explained on the basis of the clinical studies of Johnson et al. (1952) from the Mayo Clinic who observed that abnormalities of vasomotor and sudomotor function may be disassociated by lesions (chordotomies) in the antero-lateral columns of the spinal cord.

It is the author's contention therefore that disturbances of sweating and penile erection may be co-existent and may both be due to abnormalities involving the lateral horns of the dorso-lumbar cord or their connections.

It will be recalled that variation in sexual potency occurred in 4 subjects between the years of 1965 and 1966; these variations were closely accompanied by changes in patterns of sweating suggesting that these two abnormalities did not occur fortuitously.

An explanation must be offered for the changes observed in the normally potent male in 1965 who despite a conversion to a partially impotent state, showed a normal sweating pattern. This subject was analgesic below the costal margins down to the feet, suggesting an abnormality of the spino-thalamic tracts located above the mid-dorsal region. It is possible that this man did not have a lesion of the lateral horns or their connecting pathways, which would be a prerequisite for co-existing abnormalities of erection and sweating.

The author has previously observed empirically that some partially impotent individuals with MS responded favourably to parenteral treatment with testosterone propionate. A deficiency of circulating testosterone was therefore considered a possibility. If this were true, an increase in the gonadotrophin excretion in the urine could be expected. For this reason, the urinary gonadotrophin (FSH and ICSH) levels of 31 patients were assayed by Dr. G.W. Pennington in a study using 2 immature mice for each estimation (*Brown* 1955). These assays were performed prior to the introduction of the international units based on the 2nd International Reference Preparation. As the results tend to vary widely for the different ages of men (Table 4), only values in excess of 70 mouse-units were arbitrarily considered as abnormal. It should be pointed out that the gonadotrophin levels did not exceed 60 mouse-units in any normal man below the age of 50 years which upper limit, incidentally, was not exceeded by any patient under investigation.

Despite the criticisms that may be made of the gonadotrophin assay method and the author's arbitrary selection of the upper limit of normality, the results obtained were felt to be of sufficient interest to merit reporting in the hope that confirmation will be sought by others.

The urinary gonadotrophin levels are shown in Table 5. It will be evident that all the other normally potent men excreted gonadotrophins within normal limits except for the patient with mumps-orchitis. On the other hand, 37 per cent of the partially impotent individuals and approximately 66 per cent of the totally impotent subjects had abnormally elevated gonadotrophins in the urine. The small number of subjects in the 3 groups of men precluded a satisfactory statistical evaluation of the results but these findings do suggest that a deficiency in circulating testosterone exists.

Kuntz (1919) experimentally denervated the testes of dogs and demonstrated profound degenerative changes within the germinal epithelium which he believed were due to disturbances of the blood supply of the testis. *Mitchell* (1935) later found that the nerve supply of the human testis consisted of lumbar sympathetic nerve fibers. Testicular atrophy may be observed in patients with MS (*Bors et al.* 1950, *Cooper et al.* 1950, *Vas* 1966) even in the absence of either local infection, physical abnormality or systemic disease. This clinical association may be due to an abnormality of lumbar sympathetic function which might also result in both abnormalities of sweating and impairment of testosterone production by the interstitial cells of Leydig. *Simpson* (1959) has stated that testosterone can maintain spermatogenesis and penile erection in males with a deficient production of the hormone. Recently, *Hart* (1967) studied the effects of testosterone on the sexual reflexes of rats whose thoracic cords were divided. He reported that the hormone enhanced reflex erection and that withdrawal of testosterone resulted in a pronounced decline in the total number of erections induced in those animals during the observation periods. It is therefore possible that a similar situation might prevail in human subjects with MS or other spinal cord lesions. Thus, the administration of testosterone might be of therapeutic value in the management of impotent patients with spinal cord disease.

The scrotal, bulbo-cavernosus and anal sphincter reflexes are considered to be essentially autonomic in character (DeJong 1958) and mediated by the lumbosacral segments of the spinal cord. Consequently, it was thought essential that these be examined when investigating autonomic functions such as erection and sweating. The state of the autonomic reflexes is shown in Tables 6, 7 and 8. No statistical studies were undertaken because of the small numbers of patients in the various groups. Nevertheless, the results do suggest a trend. The bulbo-cavernosus and anal sphincter reflexes were present in all normally potent men but the scrotal reflexes were present in only 15 out of 17 (88%) subjects in the same group. In the partially impotent males, the reflexes appeared to be more frequently absent or doubtfully present in those individuals with elevated gonadotrophin levels in the urine as compared with those men with normal amounts of hormone excretion. Lastly, the reflexes tended to be absent in totally impotent patients. The significance of the abnormal sympathetic and parasympathetic reflexes with elevated urinary gonadotrophin excretion and disturbances of erection and sweating is not clear but the results may indicate lesions affecting the lumbar sympathetic and the sacral parasympathetic areas. It is hoped that evidence will become available in the future to explain these preliminary findings.

A few certain conclusions may be drawn from the data presented in this report. Partially and totally impotent patients with MS have abnormal patterns of sweating probably due to the presence of lesions affecting the lateral horns or their connecting pathways in the thoracic or lumbar segments of the spinal cord.

There is evidence that disease of the central nervous system, and in particular the lumbo-sacral cord, may result in impairment of penile erection.

A deficiency of circulating testosterone has been postulated in the patients examined by the author. Indirect evidence for this view was obtained by the demonstration of elevated gonadotrophins in the urine.

It may therefore be concluded that the patients with MS investigated in this study had lesions in the dorso-lumbar cord, resulting in abnormalities of sweating and impotence in 16 men.

SUMMARY

A study of disturbances of sexual function, particularly penile erection, was undertaken in 37 patients with MS. They were divided into 3 groups: normally potent, partially impotent and totally impotent. The duration of MS, average age and severity of neurological disability was determined for each group of men. Approximately 47 per cent of males investigated appeared to have some impairment of erection even though the neurological disability was not marked.

During the course of the study, autonomic functions such as sudomotor activity and postural hypotension were investigated and the integrity of the vegetative reflexes (scrotal, bulbo-cavernosus and anal sphincter) was determined. In addition, the amount of gonadotrophins excreted in the urine was assayed in 31 subjects.

The totally impotent patients perspired normally down to the level of the waist but not below, whereas the partially impotent were seen to sweat on the face, upper limbs and trunk including the groins and the perineum but not on the lower limbs. The integrity of the post-ganglionic sympathetic fibers and the presence of sweat glands in the dry skin areas were confirmed by the administration of intradermal acetylcholine and intravenous pilocarpine.

Sexual potency was observed to remit and relapse in 4 patients with a corresponding change in the pattern of sweating.

Orthostatic hypotension was not observed in any subject.

The urinary gonadotrophin excretion was abnormally elevated in all the totally impotent men and in about one-third of the partially impotent individuals.

The autonomic lumbo-sacral reflexes tended to be absent or doubtfully present in men with elevated urinary gonadotrophins but there was no clear indication that these findings were inter-related.

It is suggested that both impotence and anhydrosis may be due to an abnormality of the lateral horns or connecting pathways in the dorso-lumbar area of the spinal cord.

REFERENCES

Bennett, P.H. and J.T. Scoll (1965): Autonomic neuropathy in rheumatoid arthritis. Ann. Rheum. Dis. 24, 161–168.

Bors, E., E.T. Engle, R.C. Rosenquist and V.H. Holliger (1950): Fertility in paraplegic males. J. Clin. Endocrinol. 10. 381–398.

Brown, P.S. (1955): The assay of gonadotrophin from urine of non-pregnant human subjects. J. Endocrinol. 13, 59–64.

Coon, J.M and S. Rothman (1940): The nature of the pilomotor response to acetylcholine; some observations on the pharmacodynamics of the skin. J. Pharmacol. exp. Ther. 68, 301–311.

Cooper, I.S., E.H. Rynearson, A.A. Bailey and C.S. McCarthy (1950): The relation of spinal cord diseases to gynecomastia and testicular atrophy. Proc. Mayo Clin. 25, 320–326.

DeJong, R.N. (1958): The neurologic examination. Hoeber-Harper. New York.

Foerster, O. (1933): The dermatomes in man. Brain 56, 1–39.

Foerster, O. (1936): Symptomatologie der Erkrankungen des Rückenmarks und seiner Wurzeln, II. Die Sympatische Seitenhornkette Bumke u. Foersters Handb. Neurol. 5, 32–56.

Gillilan, L.A. (1955): Clinical aspects of the autonomic nervous system. Churchill, London.

Guttman, L. (1931): Die Schweissekretion des Menschen in ihren Bezeihungen zum Nervensystem. Z. ges. Neurol. Psychiat. 135, 1–48.

Guttman, L. (1947): Management of quinizarin sweat test. Postgrad. Med. J. 23, 353–366.

Hart, B.L. (1967): Testosterone regulation of sexual reflexes in spinal male rats. Science 155, 1283–1284.

Head, H. and A.W. Campbell (1900): The pathology of herpes zoster and its bearing on sensory localisation. Brain 23, 353–524.

Ivers, R.R. and N.P. Goldstein (1963): Multiple sclerosis: a current appraisal of symptoms and signs. Proc. Mayo Clin. 38, 457–466.

Janowitz, H.D. and M.I. Grossman (1950): The response of the sweat glands to some locally acting agents in human subjects. J. Invest. Derm. 14, 435–458.

Johnson, D.A., G.M. Roth and M.C. Winchell (1952): Autonomic pathways in the spinal cord. J. Neurosurg. 9, 599–605.

Johnson, R.H., G.J. Lee, D.R. Oppenheimer and J.M.K. Spalding (1966): Autonomic failure with orthostatic hypotension due to intermediolateral column degeneration. Quart. J. Med. 35, 276–292.

Kinsey, A.C., W.B. Pomeroy and C.E. Martin (1948): Sexual behaviour in the human male. Saunders, Philadelphia.

Kuntz, A. (1946): The autonomic nervous system. Bailliere. Tindall & Cox. London.

Kuntz, A. (1919): The innervation of the gonads of the dog. Anat. Rec. 17, 203–219.

Kurtzke, J.F. (1961): On the evaluation of disability in multiple sclerosis. Neurology (Minneap.) 11, 686–694.

List, F.L. and M.M. Peet (1938): Sweat secretion in man (1) Sweating responses in normal persons. Arch. Neurol. Psychiat. (Chic.) 39, 1228–1237.

Lumsden, C.E. (1966): Personal communication.

Masters, W.H. and V.E. Johnson (1966): Human Sexual Response, Churchill. London.

Mitchell, G.A.G. (1935): The innervation of the kidney, ureter, testicle and epididymis. J. Anat. LXX, 10–32.

Richter, C.P. and B.G. Woodruff (1945): Lumbar sympathetic dermatomes in man determined by the electrical skin-resistance method. J. Neurophysiol. 8, 323–338.

Root, W.S. and P. Bard (1947): The mediation of feline erection through sympathetic pathways with some remarks on the sexual behaviour after deafferentation of the genitalia. Amer. J. Physiol. 151, 80–90.

Rothman, S. and J.M. Coon (1939): Pilomotor action of nicotine; new pharmaco-dynamic test of skin. Arch. Derm. Syph. (Chic.) 40, 999–1000.

Semans, J.H. and O.R. Langworthy (1938): Observations on neurophysiology of sexual function in male cats. J. Urol. 40, 826–846.

Simpson, S.L. (1959): Major Endocrine disorders. Oxford Univ. Press. London.

Vas, C.J. (1966): Unpublished personal observations.

Zeitlin, A.B., T.L. Cottrell and F.A. Lloyd (1957): Sexology of the paraplegic male. Fertility & Sterility 8, 337–344.

6

Sexual Problems of the Arthritic

GEORGE E. EHRLICH, M.D.

Arthritis as a term covers a multitude of disorders. The majority of forms of arthritis are not really diseases, but are mechanical afflictions of the joints provoking the customary inflammatory responses. These are redness, heat, swelling and pain, and alteration of function. When arthritis forms part of a systemic disease, additional features develop, affecting many parts of the body. From the standpoint of sexuality, arthritis is often depersonalized by the patient, as a condition involving only part of the body would be. It is then no more an encumbrance than would be a birthmark, a clubfoot, or baldness, with one important difference. Some of the symptoms produced can affect sexual response, and the condition itself might provoke psychological responses that affect self-image. But it is necessary to recognize that just because people have arthritis, they nevertheless remain people. Some will have strongly expressed sexual needs, some will not. Some will find ways to meet these needs, some will not. Some will seek out many partners, and some will relate to only one. Some will be tempted to try a variety of positions, others will persevere in a single position. Some will seek the frequent repetition of sexual encounters, others remain celibate. What this means is that the sexual orientation of the person who has a musculoskeletal disorder is not necessarily very different from that of someone who does not. However, arthritis may impose certain limitations or alterations that influence the sexual life as they do other activities of daily living.

The physical limitations are relatively easy to define, and have been the subject of some studies. The emotional aspects are in part still conjectural, but can be defined to a degree of accuracy from a wealth of anecdotal material. It therefore becomes important to recognize that a problem exists, and that a perceptive interview may uncover it. The physical examination adds further details. Even when problems are denied, the diagnosis may permit inference of some problems. Remedies exist, although they may not always prove acceptable to the patient. Denial and societal attitudes create the major barriers. The waning of Victorianism is leveling these. Sexuality is now recognized as a legitimate area for inquiry and rehabilitation. When I wrote a chapter on the subject five years ago,[1] a single medical article had previously addressed itself to the physical aspects of arthritis in sexual behavior,[2] and only three articles to the emotional features.[3-5] Since then, at least one book,[6] one pamphlet,[7] chapters in three texts,[8-10] and three other articles[11-13] have addressed the question, at least in part. While not yet a flood, these publications testify to the increasing interest in this important aspect of human behavior.

PHYSICAL CHANGES

A popular story has Adam questioning—after Eve has been created to provide him companionship—"Lord, what's a headache?" Not only the headache but also the pain in the neck, the aching back, and pain in some nether regions can serve as a pertinent defense against unwanted sexual activity. And so also the joint pains. The implication is plain, pain can result in secondary gain.

The emotional aspects of pain will be more fully considered later. Physical pain in itself, however, is a legitimate barrier to all normal activities. Most arthritic pain is not of great intensity; the few types of pain that are, such as gout, pseudogout, rheumatic fever, and some of the more obscure syndromes, are so exquisite that they limit any activity that might otherwise be attempted, often blinding the sufferer to everything but the intensity of pain. Most of these extremely pain-provoking diseases are more likely to occur in the sexually active man than in the woman. The most frequent forms of arthritis—degenerative joint disease, rheumatoid arthritis, HLA-B27-associated variants—are characterized by relatively low intensity pain sustained over a long period of time with fluctuations. It happens that these fluctuations account for increased pain as the day wears on, with the greatest severity occurring around bedtime and during the night, although some degree of pain and considerable stiffness are present for a short time upon awakening in the morning. Thus, pain itself and its unfortunate timing are counterproductive, as far as sexual activity is concerned, interfering most by distracting and dulling libido at just those periods when sexual activity is most propitious. People who have arthritis generally feel best during the later morning hours and around noon, when, on an average day, the patient or the partner may be at work, there may be children about, and interruptions—telephone, workers, deliveries, visitors—are most likely to intervene. This deprivation of privacy interferes with sexual activity no less than the increased symptoms at otherwise more fortuitous times. Since most forms of arthritis are accompanied by stiffness in the joints after any period of rest, constricted clumsy movements and unfortunate placement of limbs, all provoking pain, can quickly and mutually extinguish arousal.

It is probably fair to say that in the majority of joints, pain and stiffness are barriers to full expression of sexuality, but only become more than that depending on additional needs and desires of the arthritic sufferer or the partner. On the other hand, sexual activity can be liberating, in that it will diminish or extinguish pain for up to several hours afterward. This providential aspect of coitus serves as a reinforcement when it is recognized as such.

Mechanical impediments to sexual expression can come about from involvement of hips, knees, or back. In addition, local lesions of the genitalia or of other parts of the body used in accessory fashion in sexual behavior can also prove troublesome. The knees and the joints of the spine may, when afflicted, require a change in the usual position. Marked flexion contractures of the knees, which characterize rheumatoid arthritis but may also be seen in osteoarthritis and in the rheumatoid variants, or a deformed spine that has become more rigid in spondyloarthropathies, may interfere with the usual positions adopted. Fortunately, very painful sacral iliitis is not frequent in women, because if it were, flexion, external rotation and abduction at the hips would be interfered with, just as if the hips themselves were involved. In the missionary position, in which the couple are face to face with the man on top, the woman generally brings her hips and sacroiliac joints to the range of motion tested for in the physical examination. Afflictions of either or both sides can seriously compromise motion (Figs. 1-6).

Hip problems are therefore the major mechanical impediments to proper sexual functioning by the woman. This is particularly true when abduction contractures have developed. Unilateral contractures of this nature or fusion of the hips by surgery or disease suffice to inhibit coitus in the missionary position. Bilateral contractures or fusion may make vaginal intercourse virtually impossible in any position. In addition, they seriously interfere with perineal hygiene. Fortunately, operations to fuse the hip in arthritis are rarely performed these days; they must have been

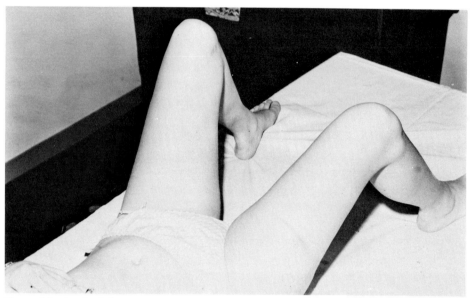

Fig. 1. Maximal abduction and external rotation which was possible for this young woman before surgical procedure at the hip relieved the associated muscle spasm and the reduced hip motion sufficiently to permit wider spread of legs. In this position, sexual intercourse would produce intolerable painful muscle cramps in the iliopsoas and other muscle groups playing on hip function.

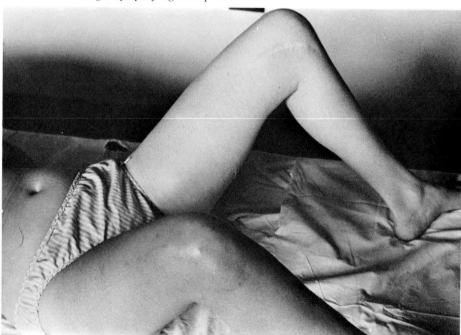

Fig. 2. Flexion, abduction and external rotation are difficult maneuvers when the hip is involved by arthritis of almost any variety. The position resulting from initiating all three maneuvers is illustrated here, and approximates the posture to be adopted in the "missionary" position by the woman. Note the scar of prior synovectomy at the left knee, necessary to permit flexion and abduction movement there.

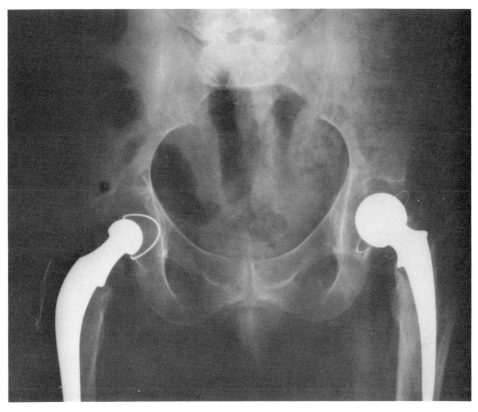

Fig. 3. Bilateral total hip replacement in a middle-aged woman whose reactive spondyl-arthropathy had severely compromised hip motion, limiting flexion and almost abolishing abduction and external rotation. Coitus was out of the question for her, and even perineal hygiene became impossible to maintain. The operative procedures here were separated by three months, although they are frequently performed simultaneously. On the left, a Charnley-Mueller prosthesis was inserted; the femoral component has a large head, and the acetabular component has a halo-like radio-opaque insert to locate it on roentgenograms. This prosthesis, and the Charnley on the right, with a different type of radio-opaque component in the acetabulum, and a smaller head as the femoral component, are cemented into the femur and ilium with methyl methacrylate bone cement. This particular Charnley prosthesis is poorly angled because the acetabular component was not correctly inserted, so motion is not as free as desired.

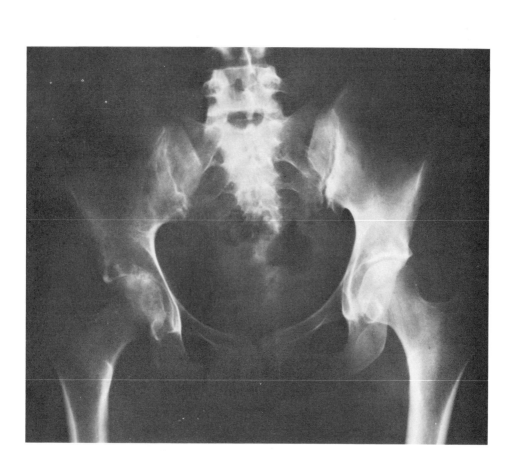

Fig. 4. Roentgenogram of the hips in which the right is severely involved in rheumatoid arthritis. Degenerative changes have also developed in the right sacroiliac joint. Pain and limitation of motion severely compromise motion of the right side, and interfere with sexual functioning.

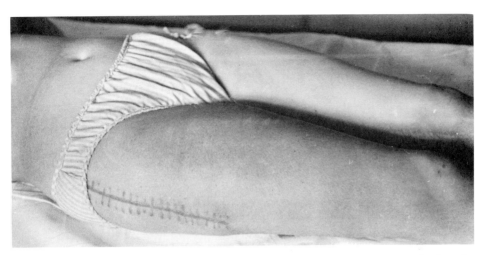

Fig. 5. For some time after surgery, the scar may be seen as a disfigurement, and might provide an aesthetic barrier in that the patient becomes shy, wondering "what others may think of" her. In time, most scars become barely visible and cease to have a psychologically deterrent effect.

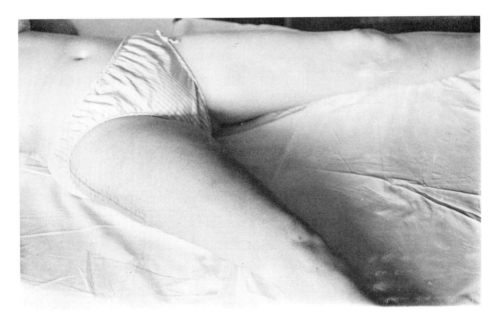

Fig. 6. Abduction of the hips was made possible only through a series of operations culminating in right total hip replacement. Progressive deterioration of a rheumatoid hip, complicated by aseptic necrosis, had finally necessitated this procedure which, until recently, was rarely performed in young persons.

particularly destructive in a former day, where the consequences upon sexual functioning were not even considered when operative intervention was decided upon. In the man, hip fusion is not quite as destructive, although it may necessitate a change in position for intercourse.

Sjögren's syndrome frequently accompanies rheumatoid arthritis and related connective tissue disorders. It tends to alter secretions of mucosal and serous glands throughout the body. It does inhibit sexual functioning, especially for the woman. Atrophic vaginitis with marked vaginal dryness is common. Natural vaginal lubrication being inhibited, dyspareunia results. Sterile lubricants may be needed to make intromission possible. Resorting to variations in sexual techniques will not necessarily help. Patients who have Sjögren's syndrome suffer from marked xerostomia which, unlike other causes of mouth dryness such as menopause, will not result in increased salivary flow upon stimulation. This symptom, plus the associated rapid dental caries often with painful gingival involvement, weighs against oral-genital activity; similarly, atrophic proctitis precludes anal intercourse. It is obvious that deformities of the fingers, poor motion of wrists, elbows and shoulders in severe rheumatoid and other major arthropathies may even prevent substitution of masturbation as a sexual outlet.

Some of the disorders with associated arthritis, such as Behcet's syndrome, Stevens-Johnson syndrome, Reiter's syndrome, and granulomatous enteritis will produce ulcerative oral and genital lesions that may be relative barriers (because of localized pain) or absolute barriers (because of aesthetic and structural deformity) (Fig. 7). The aesthetic consideration alone applies to lesions of psoriasis involving genital organs in patients who also have psoriatic arthropathy.

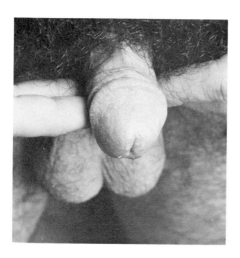

Fig. 7. Circinate balanitis and crusting at the meatus characterize Reiter's syndrome with HLA-B27 positivity. It is likely that the penile lesion will continue to trouble him for some time, perhaps recurrently or with a fixed lesion, and that from an aesthetic, if not from a functional standpoint, sexual activity may be compromised. Moreover, this lesion is associated with asymmetrical arthritis and, in this individual, ascending spondylitis which offer additional barriers to satisfactory sexual activity.

Drugs used for the treatment of arthritis may decrease sexual needs or libido. Corticosteroids are an example of the latter; actual impotence has resulted during administration to male patients, and failure to achieve an erection is one of the symptoms (complained of in circumlocution as a rule) that brings arthritic patients to their physicians. Successful corticosteroid withdrawal generally ends that problem. However, if vasculitis supervenes, the possibility of testicular atrophy also exists as one of the late consequences. Prolonged corticosteroid administration sometimes results in hypertension; drugs used in the treatment of hypertension frequently inhibit libido. So-called muscle relaxant drugs are frequently tranquilizers as well; if they are being used to reduce stiffness of muscles or joints, or to reduce the aching of fibrositis, they may also subdue libidinal impulses. It is not known if analgesic and anti-inflammatory drugs have any specific inhibitory effect, but it is known that in the majority they cross the placental barrier and thus may affect the developing fetus. Extending sexual discussion to the sometime consequence of sexual intercourse, pregnancy and its products, it is necessary to know the effects of drugs on pregnancy and even whether they are excreted in maternal milk (most are). Thus, many of these drugs may slightly increase the possibility of fetal malformation and later of hypersensitivity reactions in the infant.

EMOTIONAL FACTORS

Perhaps of more importance than the mechanical interference with sexual expression, the emotional effects of having arthritis can be devastating. The exact effects, however, depend on multiple factors and are imperfectly interpreted on the basis of anecdotal data collection.

Depression

Pain is a depressant. At the same time, some pain may be either the result or the expression of depression. In the former category there is the chronic pain of arthritis, which just never seems to let up. It becomes increasingly harder to bear. Those who have arthritis look about them and see others who are seemingly without symptoms. When encumbered by a physical disability, one longs for freedom of motion, which seems so effortless in comparison. The ultimate result of such frustration can well be rage, hostility and depression. Rage and hostility may be turned against the sexual partner as well as the family, in which case they are totally disruptive and serve to alienate. Isolation results, an isolation that the locomotion and transportation problems of the arthritic sufferer begin and that the personality alterations embellish. The unacceptability of turning rage and hostility against the family often serve to divert it to the health professional attending the patient. If this occurs, the patient's medical care will suffer, and this too may produce interferences with sexual expression because of the worsening of some symptoms left unattended. The formidable negative reaction to the patient by the family, whose tolerance of invalidism extends just so far, and by the partner, who may withdraw all sexual approaches out of compassion or counter-hostility, serves to diminish the opportunities for sexual expression even more.

Self-Image

The arthritic patient has legitimate concerns about appearance. When rheumatoid arthritis of a polyarticular variety begins in childhood, it frequently leaves the patient with short neck, recessive chin, ungainly malocclusion of the jaws and exaggerated leg length discrepancies, often accompanied by unattractive deformities of hands (Fig. 8) and feet, swayback posture, and waddling gait. When every newsstand or kiosk features pictures of handsome men and beautiful women, not just in magazines designed to appeal to eroticism but in fashion and news magazines, the patient may well compare himself or herself unfavorably with those pictured. Never mind that the majority of us cannot meet these idealized standards; the person who has a disorder sees it as a disability, whose social consequences are the handicap. The resultant withdrawal from potential sexual encounters for fear of being rejected assures that handicap, at least in the sexual sphere. In a few documented cases, satyriasis or nymphomania have developed as an obvious attempt to disprove this handicap.

Corticosteroids, used in the treatment of arthritis in many instances (not always correctly), will in time produce secondary features that also alter appearance. These include rounded moon face, trunkal obesity

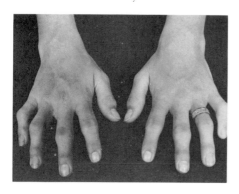

Fig. 8. Hands of an adolescent girl who suffered from polyarticular juvenile rheumatoid arthritis from the age of 6. Note the broadening of the wrists, the shortening of the hand itself with a certain spade-like appearance, and the fingers and thumb deformities that remind one of the deformities seen commonly in women of middle-age who have osteoarthritic changes. All of these are sequelae of juvenile polyarticular rheumatoid arthritis.

producing a buffalo hump and associated with thin extremities, ecchymoses, acneiform eruption, increased hairiness, cataracts, and in some instances peripheral gangrene. Corticosteroid-accelerated osteoporosis may predispose to spontaneous fractures or fractures after relatively minor trauma. One of our patients fractured an imperfectly healed osteotomy site of the distal femur during orgasm; delayed healing and osteoporosis, both corticosteroid-related, predisposed to this unusual complication. While these corticosteroid-induced deformities, on top of the arthritis, are at times disfiguring, we did see one patient who continued to take her birth control pills throughout a long siege of harrowing complications, some virtually life-threatening. This unusual case is in contrast to the majority of instances in which corticosteroid-induced alterations in appearance act to the patient's disadvantage.

Other drugs used for the treatment of some forms of arthritis can also leave their mark. Immunosuppressive drugs may cause hair loss and baldness. Wigs can be worn, of course, but attractive hair plays an important role in a woman's self-identification. Cyclophosphamide, one of these immunosuppressant drugs, can produce serious cystitis. All of these drugs can produce mouth ulcers and genital ulcers as a consequence. This is also true for gold compounds, frequently used to treat progressive rheumatoid arthritis.

The diseases themselves produce deformities. Rheumatoid arthritis generally results in flexion contractures of joints, leading not only to ungainly appearance but also to ungainly motion (Fig. 9). Painful instability of major joints is a potential sequel, necessitating the wearing of braces that may serve as formidable armor against casual sexual encounter. Likewise, the degenerative joint diseases (osteoarthrosis, osteoarthritis) lead to bony overgrowth at the joint margins producing knobby deformities, gnarled fingers, and ultimate instability. Ankylosing spondylitis and its variants result in a stiffened spine and frequently in dorsal kyphosis. Systemic lupus erythematosus may be accompanied by atrophic malar skin eruption and erythematous eruptions of the skin over other parts of the body. In progressive systemic sclerosis, ulcerations of the skin and loss of skin appendages, including hair follicles, produce unattractive deformities. In myositis, muscle strength and bulk are lost. If all this does not give a patient a negative self-image or at least create some doubts as to how the person is viewed, then one still has to take into account the way the expected partner views the patient. There may be compassion, there may be fear of hurting, but the patient may also be perceived as less attractive as time goes by. While appearance is obviously not the only factor holding marriage or sexual relationships together, it may be a factor, and lesser problems have sundered bonds. The natural fatigue that overcomes the person with

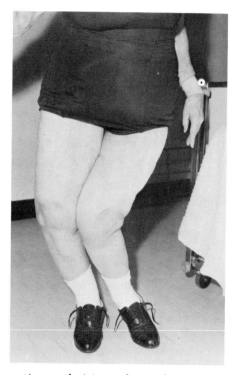

Fig. 9. Severe osteoarthritis of an erosive nature can produce grotesque deformities. While genu varum is usually associated with osteoarthritis, as seen in the right lower extremity, genu valgum may also occur, as on the left. It is obvious that hip motion must also be compromised when there is such severe knee involvement, and that from the standpoint of appearance and function, the patient's participation in sexual activity is seriously compromised.

active arthritis early in the day may be misinterpreted by the partner as a "put-off." The complaints may become intolerable and may be interpreted as substituting for the proverbial headache as an attempt to avoid sexual relations.

Finally, the patient's self-image may be wholesome, and the partner may view the patient favorably. Favorable conjunction does not assure that the patient will not interpret the partner as viewing the patient unfavorably. Little problems will be magnified. The partner's concern not to hurt may be interpreted by the patient as an aversion, a withdrawal from the sexual situation. As these problems grow, they can ultimately prove disruptive.

The enforced separation produced by hospitalization in our society does not help the matter either. A short period of separation may well be tolerable, and may even have salutary effects. It helps to serve as a "vacation" of partners from each other. A prolonged hospitalization is much like a jail sentence, however. The separation is absolute, the lack of privacy in most hospitals imposes barriers to intimacy, and the long period needed to achieve recovery from multiple surgical procedures or for a rehabilitation program in the more severely arthritic patient gives the partner outside the hospital ample opportunity for surrogate sexual partners. Marriage can be shattered on the rock of hospitalization. Separation serves as an encouragement to infidelities, and we have even discovered some developing within the hospital by the hospitalized partner and other patients.

Deprivation and the inability to enact the expected role further hampers sexual functioning, as they do any functioning. But the consequence upon sexual functioning is potentially greater, since significant alterations in lifestyle may develop. That the effect may occasionally be aphrodisiac is unexpected, although Montaigne averred "that he does not know Venus in her perfect sweetness who has not lain with a cripple."[14]

Psychogenic rheumatisms can simulate arthritis. Pure psychogenic rheumatism, sometimes called pure fibrositis, implies that no underlying organic musculoskeletal disease is present; superimposed psychogenic rheumatism (functional overlay) implies that symptoms are magnified out of proportion to the underlying lesion; residual psychogenic rheumatism (functional prolongation) implies the continuation of symptoms after organic justification has been lost.[15] All of these resemble the stiffness and pain that accompany rheumatoid arthritis, and therefore serve as potential physical barriers although they are responses to emotional problems in the main. The enormous secondary gain of being able to substitute *disease* for *unwillingness* is incalculable. The musculoskeletal disease thus becomes the implicated bystander in a more basic adjustment problem that, in itself, has nothing to do with arthritis or musculoskeletal disorders. A truism we confirmed in our studies is that if the arthritic patient hates the sexual partner, it isn't an *arthritis* problem, but rather a *psychological* problem. Successful treatment of musculoskeletal disease does not necessarily serve as a sexual restorant.

TREATMENT

The most sensible treatment consists of first recognizing the importance of sexual behavior, orientation and performance in human life. Of course there will be some to whom sex is unimportant, and arthritis does not necessarily make a difference here. There are others for whom sexual functioning is all-important, and arthritis may never be given the opportunity to interfere even if ingenious variations must first be developed. But for the vast majority of people, arthritis adds an additional problem to the problems of adjustment that all of us face.

Recent sexual attitude reassessment courses have helped the health professionals to be more at ease with patients and thus to obtain better sexual histories as part of the total anamnesis. The Victorian barriers have fallen enough so that patients, even elderly ones, are willing to discuss the matter and to accept counseling. The physical examination provides an obvious opportunity for follow-up questions about sexuality, and particularly while the range of motion of hips and the back is being assessed. If tenderness is found in any joints, a direct question may be possible regarding the effect of pain in sexual functioning. Patients today are often relieved to have the matter brought to light.

Coital activities are exertional, and therefore require the same types of preparation that obtain for other physical exertions, such as athletic endeavors. Application of moist heat in some form is usually needed for the latter, and it is often needed for sexual encounters as well. Heat is sedative to the muscles, relaxes them, and diminishes pain while increasing the range of motion. Some simple warming-up exercises may also be useful. The argument that spontaneity is lost is a legitimate one, but it should be pointed out that great harm may come to the sexual relationship if there is no physical preparation, and that the preparatory period should be viewed positively as one of heightening anticipation. Perhaps the partner can be enlisted to help in these preparatory activities, and they can serve as a type of foreplay. The tenderness of such activity may serve to enhance the relationship.

Moist heat helps in some instances; cold applications in others. Whichever has proved more beneficial should be employed. Exercises should also help prepare the afflicted areas before sexual activity. Most of these will be nonweight-bearing, range of motion exercises. It may be necessary to take analgesic or anti-inflammatory medications some thirty minutes to one hour beforehand. Timing of sexual encounters may be important, and a matinee may be preferred to early morning, night or evening hours, when pain, stiffness and fatigue may be at their height. Counseling should be offered concerning timing and position, and even to assure partners that sexual relations would not prove harmful (if that can legitimately be claimed, as it can in most instances; there are few instances when sexual relations can be harmful, and these are easily identified. One such instance is the postoperative period after total hip replacement surgery. Variable periods of abstinence from sexual intercourse exceeding a month are usually advocated. Other forms of sexual activity can, of course, be substituted). Counseling should also be provided regarding marriage, pregnancy and delivery. While these are consequences of sexual behavior, specific approaches are outside the present discussion.

Successful treatment of arthritis often removes some of the barriers to proper sexual functioning; contemporary total joint replacement arthroplasties have proved their worth in advanced stages of arthritis. Lesions associated with arthritis must be controlled symptomatically if treatment of the underlying disease is unsuccessful in removing them; advising sterile surgical lubricant for vaginal lubrication in Sjögren's syndrome, as previously mentioned, is an obvious example (petroleum jelly should be avoided, as it may encourage infection).

To counsel most effectively, the health professional needs to understand the sexual functioning pattern of the individual. Earlier studies have shown that the premorbid frequency of sexual encounters was the best guide to the subsequent behavior, so any history must explore the frequency of intercourse, satisfaction achieved by the partners, variations in positions used and willingness to try others, and the ability to discuss the sexual problems with the partner. Other questions will obviously grow out of these, and the patient's assessment of the psychosocial factors and any potential ethical problems related to variance of sexual practice is important. The type of contraceptive used is also important; an arthritic man with disabling arthritis in his fingers may find it impossible to put on a condom sheath; a woman may inexpertly insert a diaphragm. Oral hormonal contraceptives used by many women can predispose to thrombosis, already a potential complication of rheumatic diseases or their treatment, especially in patients having a previously demonstrated increased tendency to platelet aggregation. Tenderness and companionship must be stressed in counseling. Variations in sexual position can be discussed, especially those that do not require weight-bearing by afflicted joints or a range of motion beyond the capability of the arthritic joint.

RESULTS OF COUNSELING

The results are astonishing. Our addition of sexual history, usually obtained by the rehabilitation nurse specialist in the arthritis center inpatient unit, to the total work-up has released floodgates and amazing enthusiasm in those questioned. Even elderly women with rather rigid backgrounds, who might be expected to cavil at answering the questions, have demonstrated their delight that the subject was brought up. Often they will exclaim, "Why has no one asked before?" Counseling is generally well received. An occasional patient rejects the variant positions; one such patient was a 19-year-old married woman from a rural coal-mining area, who, with her husband, held fairly Fundamentalist beliefs and rejected any but the missionary position, which she was totally incapable of maintaining because of severe hip involvement. Ultimately, bilateral hip surgery led to a satisfactory resumption of the sexual relationship, which in fact was restarted in her hospital room when her husband came to take her home—to the consternation of the nurses and the delight of some of the other patients!

Many patients are not so fortunate. Those who live in retirement communities, often alone because of the death of the mate, often find it difficult to seek out new partners. This is particularly true for women, who the life tables tell us survive to later years than men, and who because of fear of disapproval by grown children or because of more restricted backgrounds (as well as a shortage of potential male partners) will not enter into new sexual relationships easily. However, one of the gratifying aspects of resumed sexual activity related by the majority of patients is the beneficial effect of coitus upon pain. Symptoms may well be relieved for up to 6 to 8 hours following sexual activity.

Several illustrative cases dramatize the interplay between arthritis and sexual behavior:

1) A 58-year-old woman had developed Heberden's nodes and other minor stigmata of interphalangeal osteoarthritis some seven years previously. Her lesions had never been particularly symptomatic after an initial inflammatory onset. She required no specific treatment, and only consulted her physician episodically. The era of new permissiveness had brought variations in sexual positions to the husband's attention. Several years older than his wife, and just as primly brought up, he suggested to her that their sexual relations had always borne the aura of sameness, and asked her to fondle his penis, something she had never done before. When she complied, he then asked her to perform fellatio, to which she agreed. The next morning, she awoke with severe pain in her hands and extremely stiff fingers. This was the seeming onset of her rheumatoid arthritis which progressed to crippling, necessitating many reconstructive operative procedures and becoming seropositive accompanied by Sjögren's syndrome. Not until the sexual interview did this woman reveal this story and express the belief shared with her husband that the masturbatory and oral activity, both against their Fundamental religious beliefs, had somehow created the arthritis that followed immediately with all of its associated signs. Although she and her husband were still devoted to each other, their sexual relationship had virtually ceased that fateful evening.

2) Another patient, a middle-aged woman, was in such a hurry to resume long-delayed sexual activity that it was the first thing she did on arriving home after bilateral total hip surgery, which had been preceded by an osteotomy of the lower end of the femur. Unfortunately, her orgasmic contraction was so intense that she fractured her femur through the osteotomy site. She was forced to return to the hospital with an inevitable postponement of gratification. The story was only later discovered; the original tale had it that she fell on her way to the bathroom in the dark. Perhaps the fact that she was not married led to this prevarication.

3) A young woman in her early 20's, not particularly popular, met and married a somewhat constrained young man shortly after developing relatively mild and seemingly easily controllable rheumatoid arthritis. During her subsequent pregnancy, she lost all symptoms and signs of her disease. Six months after the birth of her son, rheumatoid arthritis recurred. It is a well known fact that pregnancy often leads to a remission of rheumatoid arthritis and that delivery is followed by exacerbation in many instances. When the sequence occurred here, she withdrew sexually from her husband, fearful that intercourse would mean pregnancy, and pregnancy would be followed by worsening of her disease. A divorce soon followed. While some basic adjustment difficulties are highlighted by this case, arthritis served as a pretext for cessation of all sexual activity.

4) A sexually vigorous married truck driver, 37 years of age, developed rheumatoid arthritis. His physician prescribed increasingly larger doses of corticosteroids. Although he was able to continue working fitfully, he was increasingly disabled by his disease, markedly fatigued, and often incapable of driving the truck. In the interview, he equated his truck driving with his masculinity. To preserve the latter, he had to be able to accomplish the former. The large doses of corticosteroids were thought to be necessary to assure his continued ability to work. Unfortunately, they also contributed to impotence; reduced libido is a frequent complication of corticosteroid therapy. A subsequent hospitalization in the Arthritis Center initiated corticosteroid withdrawal and institution of remittive therapy. Rheumatoid arthritis abated, and he resumed driving a truck; shortly thereafter, he was again able to boast of his sexual prowess.

5) A young man in his late 20's had suffered from Reiter's syndrome with complicating spondylitis-like changes since the age of 19. He had contracted urethritis and conjunctivitis while on military duty in the Pacific, following his first sexual exposure. He had been the only child of a widowed mother to whom he had been quite close, and who had brought him up in a religious home; sexual transgression represented sin to him, and he saw the triple complex of urethral, conjunctival, and joint disease as retribution. He became progressively crippled with extremely stiff joints, ultimately being almost unable to walk except with the aid of two canes and a shuffling propelled gait. In one of his rehabilitation hospitalizations, he found himself in a room with another young man who had severe fulminant systemic lupus erythematosus and a sociopathic personality. He became friendly with this man, who was separated from his wife, and took him into his home after they were both discharged from the hospital. The critically ill patient was able to get around much better than the patient with Reiter's syndrome, and was thus able to do the shopping and help maintain the household. In re-

turn, the young patient who had Reiter's syndrome was able to provide a paid-for home, a car and companionship. His new friend was soon hospitalized with acute cerebritis and died in the intensive care unit of a strange hospital. The widow came to get his effects from the apartment, at which time the patient met her for the first time. She was a very attractive young woman, and he found himself drawn to her.

For the first time since the episode of "venereal" disease that began his invalidism, this young man found an object for his sexual attentions outside himself. His intervening ten years had been spent masturbating and fantasizing. He began to court the young woman actively and found her somewhat responsive. They had no sexual relationship, as he was incapable of moving appropriately, and she really served to supplant her former husband as his companion. However, plans went ahead for marriage. In interviews, it was clear that for our patient, she represented fulfillment and stability, and that his sexual attention had not been markedly aroused as yet. She found many reasons for avoiding an interview, but it was clear that her interest was chiefly in having herself and her two children supported, for which she was willing to keep a household.

The patient finally decided that more could be done for him than he had permitted in the past, and he returned to the hospital for bilateral total hip replacement arthroplasties and other measures designed to make it possible for him to move better. During this hospitalization, he also began to realize that he was sexually attracted to his new wife, and that he was eagerly looking forward to discharge from the hospital to assert his marital rights. The closer to discharge the time came, the more excited he became, and the less his wife seemed to visit. She found all manner of excuses for avoiding the hospital, and it was clear to the staff that she was becoming increasingly terrified. It seemed that she had married her first husband during his illness, and her current husband during a major illness, and it was obvious that in both cases she chose invalided men to avoid sexual relationships. Clearly, what had started as an asexual companionship with her current husband was turning into a threatening situation. Just before he was to be discharged from the hospital, feverishly anticipating the consummation of his marriage, he learned that his wife had been hospitalized in a psychiatric hospital. She had had a complete breakdown, was totally withdrawn in a schizophrenic episode and, as it subsequently turned out, needed to remain hospitalized with severe psychotic symptoms. Clearly the threat of a sexually active husband was more than she had bargained for, and this had precipitated her collapse. For our patient, this episode provoked considerable depression and indecision about his future sexual identification and course. He returned to his home to think things over, even though an ambitious rehabilitation program went begging through its abrupt change of direction.

6) A 19-year-old woman had developed polyarticular juvenile rheumatoid arthritis at age 8. The disease had become inactive at age 15, but had left her with a 3-inch shortening of the left lower extremity, and with short stubby hands and feet. By contemporary standards, she was moderately unattractive in appearance, but her personality was very pleasant and well adjusted. She became engaged to a young man who worked as a skilled laborer and was of similar background and whose health had always been good. His family strongly objected to the proposed marriage because of the girl's deformities. Despite these objections, the marriage took place, but his family was not in attendance. The couple settled into a reasonably adjusted marriage, and at last reports, had two healthy children, both born by cesarian section because of the woman's contracted pelvis, part of the stigmata of her juvenile rheumatoid arthritis.

7) Another young woman, also aged 19, had developed juvenile rheumatoid arthritis at age 11. Her disease continued to smolder and was only partially controlled through continued administration of injections of gold compounds. There were relatively minor changes in the hands and feet, chiefly characterized by short stubby digits and poor ability to close her hand, thus precluding good grasp and good strength. She had the recessive chin and short neck characteristic of polyarticular juvenile rheumatoid arthritis in many patients. By contemporary standards, she was actually more attractive than the young woman who had married successfully. However, she regarded herself as ugly because of her rheumatoid deformities, and was chronically moderately depressed. She never dated, and turned down all requests for dates or invitations to parties where she was likely to be in mixed company. She led a lonely life and commented that obviously no man would want her, and if he did, it would be only for a temporary sexual release if no one else was available.

8) A third young woman, also aged 19, had developed juvenile rheumatoid arthritis of a polyarticular nature at age 10. She still required treatment with injections of gold compounds and supplementation with non-steroidal anti-inflammatory compounds. While her disease was usually under control, there were occasional flare-ups. She had taken brief courses of corticosteroids to relieve the symptoms during such flares. She was obese, had shortened hands and feet, a slight leg length discrepancy, and contractures of both elbows. Her neck was short, her chin only slightly recessive. Her social life was characterized by sexual promiscuity, and she was willing to take on as many as eight men consecutively. Her sexual initiation was at age 12, shortly after her acute

onset of disease came under control, when she was known to the boys in her neighborhood as someone who was always available upon payment of chewing gum, candy or, at times, no payment at all. The neighborhood boys described her as a "pig" and used her as a masturbatory substitute. Psychological evaluation disclosed that she took on this role to provide constant reinforcement of her sexual identity and, as she saw it, of her desirability, something that her mirror failed to reflect.

All three women came from similar backgrounds, in the same neighborhood. All three had had religious upbringings, had attended parochial schools, were first-generation Americans, and had vaguely known each other, although they moved in different social circles. Factors other than juvenile rheumatoid arthritis obviously played some role; placement in the family, the number of older or younger siblings, the attitude of the parents, and differing attitudes of the nuns who were their teachers. Nonetheless, in all three instances, juvenile rheumatoid arthritis played a significant part in their development and colored their lives, and their social and sexual behavior was colored by this chronic illness.

9) A young woman in a rural community developed juvenile rheumatoid arthritis at age 13. A recessive chin developed rather rapidly, but plastic surgery restored the contours of the chin, albeit somewhat asymmetrically. The hands and feet, through early closure of epiphyses and absorption of bone, were short and pudgy. A marked swayback deformity developed, and a waddling gait because of bilateral severe hip involvement. Even before multiple surgical procedures that reduced the swayback deformity gave her a normal gait through total hip replacements, and permitted better hand function through wrist and metacarpophalangeal surgery and better foot function through total ankle arthroplasty, she had lived a relatively well-adjusted life, had completed secretarial courses and worked full-time, driving herself to and from work, a total of 16 miles each day in the process. She steadily dated one man who lived in her community, and she and her friend both were members of well-regarded families who enjoyed higher socioeconomic status in their town. In an effort to draw attention away from her ungainly hands and feet, she was given to wearing tight sweaters that emphasized her buxom figure. she was always well-groomed, her hair bleached blond, set in a Marilyn Monroe style, and interviews confirmed that her self-image and sexual identification had compensated for her deformities; she considered herself quite attractive, and her friend thought of her as attractive as well.

10) Another young woman developed polyarticular juvenile arthritis which continued to flare-up at various joints producing acute synovitis. However, no structural deformities developed. Except for occasional

stiffness that precluded normal gait at those times, she developed into a rather attractive young woman. Her self-image was poor, however, and she shunned social contact. Hip involvement led to poor abduction and external rotation of the hips. She had had a strict upbringing and her moral code prohibited sexual experimentation. She accepted the arthritis in the hips as a welcome physical barrier that kept her from "sinful behavior." A number of operative procedures were performed ultimately to permit freer motion of her joints. She is fully employed, but suffers spells of depression, is under psychiatric care, and cannot see herself as others see her. She thinks she is quite unattractive, and she shuns even casual dating; her psychosexual development is retarded at a prepubescent level.

11) A young man, now age 23, developed juvenile rheumatoid arthritis at age 8 and was treated with corticosteroids. His height is foreshortened and his hands stubby but quite functional. Because he is only 5 feet tall and in appearance like a boy of 13, he has denied himself sexual dating relationships. He has sublimated by having female friends whom he talks to, writes poetry to, and cooks for, but he otherwise intellectualizes his sexual life.

12) A woman developed an acute illness of which arthritis was a component. Severe pulmonary involvement led to lobectomy. She developed thrombosis of the iliac veins, necessitating inferior vena cava plication. Subsequently, she developed superior vena cava thrombosis with obstruction. Recurrent crops of mouth ulcers, erythema nodosum, and vaginal ulcers permitted labelling of the disease as Behcet's syndrome. The mucocutaneous lesions significantly interfered with sexual relations with her husband. He began a strenuous exercise program as a form of sublimation, avoided sexual contact with his wife and, when the serious complicating lesions of the major veins and lung developed, withdrew from her for fear, as he put it, that if he touched her he might kill her. Marital discord developed, and he took the children with him when he separated from his wife while she was undergoing prolonged treatment in the hospital.

These cases illustrate the complexities of sexual adjustment as part of lifestyle alterations in which rheumatic diseases play a greater or lesser part. They derive from interviews by a trained staff.

Our rehabilitation nurse and psychologists use personal interviews and group discussions, film strips and pamphlets to ferret out problems and to counsel. A psychiatrist is available for discussion and treatment of the more severe problems. Patients and their "significant others" are encouraged to participate in sexual awareness reassessment programs offered to groups at our rehabilitation center. The physicians become involved in case detection and counseling, first also undergoing training to disabuse them of preconceived erroneous ideas and to make them less uncomfortable in such discussions.

Not every health professional is yet comfortable in discussing sexual behavior with patients, nor is every patient ready for such a discussion. Embarrassment and inhibitions must be overcome, preferably through desensitizing courses rather than by sweeping the problem under the rug, ignoring it, or worse, giving inadequate, inaccurate or biased advice based on prejudice rather than on knowledge. Through the efforts of a few dedicated individuals, sexuality is taking its place among the activities of daily living for people of all ages and sexes. Arthritis—being more a condition than a disease—should therefore not alter this truth. The discussion should be in words the examiner/counselor and patient are both comfortable with for maximal benefit to be achieved. Relevant prognostic implications should not be avoided and, if raised by the professional, can greatly increase the success rate of all of the treatment offered, since it will be interpreted as perspicacity by the patient.

Is it not as important to help the patient achieve better sexual functioning as it is to improve any of the other aspects of daily life that arthritis and other musculoskeletal disorders threaten?

ACKNOWLEDGMENTS

Mary P. Brassell, R.N., B.S., and Philip Spergel, Ed.D., conducted the sexual interviews and counseling sessions in the Arthritis Center at Moss Rehabilitation Hospital on which many of the reports in this chapter are based.

REFERENCES

1. Ehrlich, G.E. Sexual Problems of the Arthritic Patient. *In* Ehrlich, G.E. (Ed.) Total Management of the Arthritic Patient. Philadelphia, J.B. Lippincott, 1973.
2. Currey, H.L.F. Osteoarthritis of the hip joint and sexual activity. Ann. Rheum. Dis. 29:488, 1970.
3. Fink, S.L., Skipper, J.K. and Hallenbeck, P.N. Physical disability and problems in marriage. J. Marriage Family 38:64, 1968.
4. Ford, A.B. and Orfirer, A.P. Sexual behavior and the chronically ill patient. Med. Aspects Human Sexuality 1:51, 1967.
5. Sadoughi, W., Leshner, M. and Fine, H.L. Sexual adjustment in the chronically ill and physically disabled population: A pilot study. Arch. Phys. Med. 52:311, 1971.
6. Heslinger, K. Not Made of Stone. The Sexual Problems of Handicapped People. Leyden-Noordhoff International Publishing, 1974.
7. Arthritis and Rheumatism Council, United Kingdom: Marriage, Sex and Arthritis.

8. Blau, S.P. and Schultz, D. How to Cope with the Question of Sex and Arthritis. *In* Arthritis: Complete Up-to-Date Facts for Patients and Their Families. Garden City, N.Y., Doubleday, 1974.
9. Katz, W.A. Sexuality and Arthritis. *In* Katz, W.A. (Ed.) Rheumatic Diseases. Diagnosis and Management. Philadelphia, J.B. Lippincott, 1977.
10. Swinburn, W.R. Sexual Counselling for the Arthritic. *In* Wright, V. (Ed.) Osteoarthrosis. Clinics in the Rheumatic Diseases 2/2. Philadelphia, W.B. Saunders, 1976.
11. Bidgood, F.E. Sexuality and the handicapped. SIECUS Report 11:2, 1974.
12. Hill, R.H. Herstein, A. and Walters, K. Juvenile rheumatoid arthritis: Follow-up into adulthood—medical, sexual and social status. Canad. Med. Assoc. J. 114:790, 1976.
13. Labby, D.H. Sexual concomitants of disease and illness. Postgrad. Med. 58:103, 1975.
14. Benedek, T. Disease as aphrodisiac. Bull. Hist. Med. 45:322, 1971.
15. Ehrlich, G.E. Psychosomatic aspects of musculoskeletal disorders. Postgrad. Med. 38:614, 1965.

7

Sexual Adjustment for Arthritic Patients

LAURO S. HALSTEAD, M.D.

For purposes of this review, arthritis includes those disease processes which produce chronic signs and symptoms in one or more joints. As with other chronic illnesses, sexual function and adjustment in persons with arthritis has been relatively ignored until recently. However, numerous reports in the literature have made it clear that sexual interest and activity continue to remain important, even for those who are wheelchair-bound and have major movement impairments.[1-3]

Satisfactory sexual adjustment in the arthritic poses the same spectrum of problems common to persons without a physical handicap. Chronic arthritis, however, presents additional problems, especially in three key areas. First, the nature of a sexual dysfunction is likely to be more difficult to diagnose since it is frequently complicated by the underlying medical condition. Second, successful intervention is more elusive because of the fluctuating physical and emotional factors often associated with arthritis. Third, as with other long-term disabilities, arthritis places special stresses on the patient's sexual partner and their relationship. Many patients report it is often easier for them than for their partner to accept limitations or explore alternative forms of sexual expression because they have had to deal more directly with the problem of coping and adapting to their disability in other areas. Thus, *involving the partner* is especially critical in assessing and managing sexual dysfunctions in arthritic patients.

HISTORY

A thorough history of sexual function and enjoyment taken with tact and candor can be therapeutic as well as diagnostic. For many patients, your sexual history may be the first any physician has ever taken. The simple fact that you are sufficiently concerned to ask questions can relieve the patient's sense of anxiety, isolation, and frustration. The following are a few practical guidelines:

1. *Take the history in an appropriate context* (e.g., during the review of systems, after inquiring about GU and GI functions, or during the physical examination).

2. *Be systematic.* Levitt[4] has proposed one approach which is comprehensive yet practical. With arthritis patients, three time periods are especially helpful to explore: sexual adjustment prior to onset of symptoms; adjustment during exacerbations; and present adjustment. Previous adjustment provides a good insight into potential outcome. Is the patient as active sexually as he or she would like to be? Has arthritis caused any change in sexual activity or satisfaction? Are there other reasons for decreased satisfaction? When did they begin?

3. *Explore feelings of loss.* Even in mild cases, most persons with physical limitations feel they have experienced a loss which affects the way they view themselves. What do they feel they have lost? Has it changed their self-image? Do they feel less masculine or feminine?

PHYSICAL EXAMINATION

Ehrlich has emphasized the importance of the "mechanical barrier" in patients, especially when there is involvement of the hip joints.[5] The FABER maneuver (an acronym for flexion, abduction, and external rotation at the hips) performed with the patient supine is helpful in identifying mechanical limitations which may interfere with coitus and often are amenable to surgery. Testing for hip and pelvic mobility presents another appropriate time to initiate questions about sexual activity and satisfaction or to raise additional questions based on physical findings.

DIAGNOSIS

In establishing a diagnosis, it is helpful to distinguish between primary and secondary sexual dysfunction. Primary dysfunction refers to a long-standing problem which has been present for most of an individual's adolescent and adult life, such as a male who has never had an erection. Patients with primary dysfunction should be referred to a specialist. Secondary dysfunction refers to problems that have a fairly recent onset, such as intermittent or situational impotence. Such patients' sexual problems may be either unrelated or related to and aggravated by arthritis. Patients with secondary dysfunction, which comprise the largest group, can often be handled quite successfully by the primary physician.

TREATMENT

The following topics and suggestions are intended principally to be of assistance in dealing with patients with secondary sexual dysfunctions. Because pain is a predominant problem in all forms of arthritis, most of the therapeutic suggestions refer to that symptom, although the principles may apply to other symptoms as well.

1. *Disease activity.* The physician should ensure that an accurate diagnosis is made of the underlying disease process and that appropriate measures are used to minimize active signs and symptoms. In a recent study of patients with juvenile rheumatoid arthritis, Hill et al. found that ongoing disease activity rather than absolute severity of disability was the major factor in preventing a satisfactory sexual adjustment.[1] It is also important that the physician rule out medications which might aggravate the sexual dysfunction, although most drugs used to treat arthritis, except for corticosteroids, do not impair libido or sexual performance.

2. *Timing.* Identify the time of day and set of circumstances when pain is consistently least severe. Suggest that the patient plan his or her sexual activity around those times. The physician should also explore altering the schedule of medications so that the period of maximum effectiveness coincides with planned sexual activity.

3. *Position.* Suggest that the patient try a variety of positions to discover which is most comfortable and requires the least expenditure of energy. Many couples have found that the side-by-side positions are the most satisfactory—either face-to-face or back-to-front—especially when spine and hip mobility are problems.

4. *Aids.* Discover what works best to relieve or reduce pain. If heat is effective, suggest that the patient take a warm bath before sexual activity, preferably with his or her partner. For the person with severe joint limitations or where repetitious movement causes discomfort, water beds and massage oils can help reduce friction and fatigue.

5. *Nonsexual activities.* Some of the best clues about what provides effective pain relief can be obtained by exploring enjoyable nonsexual activities and discovering what can be done to minimize discomfort in those situations.

6. *Partners.* Chronic illness places special demands on the nondisabled partner. Open, honest communication becomes especially impor-

tant. If possible, talk with the partner alone and then together with the patient. What is the partner's perception of the dysfunction? What are the partner's attitudes about the patient's arthritis? Is the partner as sexually active and satisfied as he or she would like to be? When the patient is severely impaired, there is often an unrecognized problem for the sex partner who also plays a major "care provider" role. Many patients have found that having a third person be the care provider at certain times relieves the partner and gives him or her more time and energy to concentrate on the sexual role.

7. *Information.* It is surprising how many myths persist about how our bodies function. A special concern of arthritic patients is whether or not certain activities will be harmful. Providing basic information about arthritis as well as the anatomy and physiology of sexual functioning can relieve unnecessary apprehension and fears.

8. *Attitudes.* For most persons, whether able-bodied or disabled, attitudes regarding sex present the largest barrier toward achieving a satisfactory sexual adjustment. Helping patients reassess their sexual attitudes can be a very effective therapeutic measure.

9. *Pain and pleasure.* Sex should be pleasurable and a source of gratification. Many patients have reported that sex can have an analgesic effect which sometimes lasts for hours. For others, however, the pain of arthritis is a more common experience than the pleasure of sex. The physician's goal is to minimize the pain of the former and enhance the pleasure of the latter.

REFERENCES

1. Hill, R.H., Herstein, A. and Walters, K. Juvenile rheumatoid arthritis: follow-up into adulthood—medical, sexual and social status. Canad. Med. Assn. J. 114:790, 1976.
2. Currey, H.L.F. Osteoarthritis of the hip joint and sexual activity. Ann. Rheum. Dis. 29:488, 1970.
3. Halstead, L.S., Halstead, M.G., Salhoot, J.T., Stock, D.D. and Sparks, R.W. Sexual attitudes, behavior and satisfaction for able-bodied and disabled participants attending workshops in human sexuality. (In press)
4. Levitt, E.E. Sexual Counseling: What the Busy Physician Can, and Cannot, Do. Postgrad. Med. 58:910, 1975.
5. Ehrlich, G.E. Total Management of the Arthritic Patient. Philadelphia, J.B. Lippincott, 1973.

8

Sexual Dysfunction in Diabetic Men

ROBERT C. KOLODNY, M.D., CHARLES B. KAHN, M.D.,

H. HOWARD GOLDSTEIN, M.D. AND DONALD M. BARNETT, M.D.

Sexual dysfunction is a common complication of diabetes mellitus in both men[1-5] and women.[6] Despite previous investigators generally agreeing that the prevalence of impotence in diabetic men approximates 50 per cent, there is controversy surrounding the etiology of this problem. Endocrine causes of the impotence associated with diabetes have been suggested[2,3] although not verified. Vascular complications of diabetes may produce impotence on the basis of large vessel disease (e.g., the Leriche syndrome) or, theoretically, secondary to microvascular changes. The neurologic factor, long felt to be important in the pathogenesis of erective difficulties in diabetic males, has been recently re-emphasized by the demonstration of a high association of neurogenic vesical abnormalities in a group of impotent diabetics.[5] Other systemic diseases, patterns of drug use, and psychological factors[7] may all contribute to difficulty in the clinical evaluation of the etiology of impotence in the diabetic male, and may confuse the choice of treatment modality.

In addition to impotence, other types of sexual dysfunction may complicate diabetes, including retrograde ejaculation[4] and premature ejaculation. This study was undertaken to obtain further information concerning sexual dysfunction in male diabetics.

METHOD

One hundred and eighty-six men between the ages of eighteen and eighty-three with previously diagnosed diabetes mellitus were interviewed during outpatient visits to Joslin Clinic during 1971. Of this group, 175 men completed all phases of this study. For each subject, a sexual and medical history was obtained, a physical examination was performed and the following laboratory studies were done: complete blood count, urinalysis, T4, 12 channel chemistry screening profile and plasma testosterone determination.[8]

The interview included specific questions regarding sexual distress; the mode of onset; duration, frequency and degree of impotence; the temporal relationship of impotence to the clinical onset of diabetes; and the current existence of such signs of intact neurovascular function as nocturnal or morning erections, or the ability to obtain an erection during masturbation. A review of the patient's medical records was also conducted to supplement the clinical material obtained in this study, including an itemization of current medications; assessment of the control of diabetes, and the presence of retinopathy, nephropathy, peripheral vascular disease, neuropathy or other diabetic complications.

RESULTS

Eighty-five of 175 diabetic men (48.6 per cent) were impotent. The age distribution among impotent diabetics and the control diabetics is shown in Table 1. In the group of men with impotence, the mean age was 53.2 years; in the control group, the mean age was 45.4 years.

TABLE 1. Age distribution of study subjects

Age	Number of subjects	Number of impotent
18-24	11	0
25-31	14	4
32-38	13	5
39-45	21	11
46-52	26	12
53-59	33	17
60-66	31	18
67-73	16	11
74-80	8	6
81 plus	2	1
Totals	175	85

There was no apparent correlation between duration of diabetes and presence or absence of impotence (see Table 2). In fourteen men, impotence had been an initial manifestation of diabetes and preceded the establishment of the diagnosis; eight of these men regained normal potency following the initiation of diabetic therapy.

Twenty-nine men reported impotence of less than one year's duration. Although these men, taken as a group, gave the impression of poorer control than a group of randomly selected, age-matched diabetic men (by review of the preceding year's medical records and laboratory tests), formal criteria assessing control had not been planned prospectively and thus no definite conclusions could be drawn.

Typically, the onset of impotence was gradual, usually progressing over a period of six months to a year with a period of time during which there was a decreased firmness of the erection but not total absence of the erectile response. However, in men with impotence of more than one year's duration, total loss of erective function was described by fifty-four of fifty-six men. Seven men (8.2 per cent) reported the relatively sudden onset of impotence. These men provided information that strongly suggested that their sexual distress was psychogenic: morning or nocturnal erections occurred frequently, the ability to masturbate was unimpaired, or a selective pattern of impotence was seen (Table 3).

TABLE 2. Characteristics of study subjects

Characteristic	Impotent (N = 85)	Not impotent (N = 90)
Mean age (years)	53.2	45.4
Duration of diabetes (years)	6.4	5.9
Treatment:		
Diet alone	1	3
Oral agents	38	43
Insulin	46	44
Complications:		
Retinopathy	19	20
Neuropathy	32	19
Nephropathy	11	10
Hypertension	10	8
Weekly coital frequency		
At present	0.1	2.0
Five years ago	1.9	2.3
Plasma testosterone	627 ± 15 (S.E.M.) ng./100 ml.	637 ± 14 (S.E.M.) ng./100 ml.

92

TABLE 3. Differential Diagnosis

Types	Libido	Erection loss	A.M. Erections	Masturbation ability
Organic (most causes)	N↓	Abrupt	Absent	Absent
Diabetes	N↑	Gradual	Absent	Partially/totally
Psychological (including aging male)	N↓	Abrupt	Present	Unimpaired

Table 2 presents additional characteristics of the impotent and non-impotent diabetic men. Mode of treatment of diabetes did not correlate with the presence or absence of impotence; insulin-requiring men with impotence were using an average daily dose of 40.4 U. while nonimpotent insulin-requiring men were using an average daily dose of 42.3 U. The incidence of vascular disease, as evidenced by retinopathy and/or nephropathy, and of hypertension was similar in the two groups. The incidence of neuropathy was significantly greater in the group of men with impotence (37.6 per cent) than in nonimpotent diabetics (21.1 per cent) ($>$ .05 using the chi-square test).[9]

The means for plasma testosterone in the impotent diabetic men (627 ± 15 ng./100 ml.) and the group without impotence (637 ± 14 ng./100 ml.) (mean ± S.E.M.) were remarkably similar. Plasma testosterone levels of the nonimpotent diabetics and all but three of the eighty-five impotent diabetics were in the normal range (400 to 1,000 ng./100 ml.). A subject with documented hemochromatosis had a plasma testosterone of 256 ng./100 ml.; a subject who was receiving estrogen therapy for carcinoma of the prostate had a plasma testosterone of 313 ng./100 ml. (in this case, impotence antedated the prostatic disease by six years); and a man with uremia (BUN = 85 mg. per cent, Hgb = 8 gm.) had a plasma testosterone of 334 ng./100 ml. The latter three subjects reported markedly depressed libido, in contrast to the normal libido described by the remainder of the men, and had small testes. Two other subjects also had small testes and impotence, but their libido and plasma testosterone levels were normal. Five men had previously been treated with testosterone with transient improvement.

Two subjects (1.1 per cent) had retrograde ejaculation and four subjects (2.3 per cent) reported premature ejaculation. No case of ejaculatory incompetence was discovered.

DISCUSSION

The frequent occurrence of impotence with diabetes mellitus described in this study (eighty-five of 175 men or 48.6 per cent) is in agreement with previous reports.[2,3,5] Despite the frequency of this disorder, the pathophysiologic mechanism resulting in loss of erective function in diabetes is unclear.

Schoffling and co-workers[3] reported in 1963 that two-thirds of their patients with impotence and diabetes had decreased urinary excretion of pituitary gonadotropin (determined by bioassay), yet urinary excretion of 17-ketosteroids was increased. According to these workers, the elevated 17-ketosteroid levels were due to an increase in adrenal androgens with low potency, while the metabolites of testosterone were decreased. In addition, they found that one-third of their group had low sperm counts. They reported that all but one of their patients aged forty or under responded significantly to therapy with a combination of chorionic gonadotropin and testosterone; most patients over age forty responded significantly to testosterone therapy alone.

In more recent work by Schoffling, thirteen of forty diabetic men with sexual disturbances were found to have low plasma testosterone levels, whereas only one of thirteen diabetic men without sexual disturbances had subnormal levels. However, the normal range described in this report is extremely narrow; using values more commonly accepted as the normal male range would show only six of these men to have diminished plasma testosterone. Although Schoffling states that "endocrine dysfunction is the main cause" of impotence in diabetes, our results weigh heavily against this view. Further documentation of the normal plasma testosterone levels of impotent diabetic men is provided by others.[5,10]

The results of testosterone therapy, alone or in common with chronic gonadotropin, have not been successful in the treatment of impotent diabetics in our experience or in the experience of Ellenberg.[5] Indeed, Schoffling's group is the only one to advocate its usefulness under these circumstances. In addition to possible adverse effects resulting from testosterone therapy such as sodium retention, hepatic dysfunction and prostatic hypertrophy, the administration of exogenous androgen may increase libido while pathologic conditions resulting in erective dysfunction are unchanged, thus creating a far less comfortable and more frustrating situation for the patient.

Ellenberg's work presents careful documentation of the importance of neuropathy in the pathogenesis of impotence in diabetic men.[5] Judging by the clinical examination alone, we detected significantly greater incidence of neuropathy in diabetic men with impotence than in nonimpotent diabetics, thus supporting the contention that impotence in diabetes is most likely due to neurogenic factors. Additionally, Weiss[11] in a review of the physiology of penile erection discusses the various anatomical sites of pathology that could account for the problem. Valve-like structures called "polsters" containing smooth muscle have been described near the corpora cavernosa and are under the control of the autonomic nervous system. Poor neural transmission most likely would disturb the steady state of increased inflow of blood into the erectile tissues. This site of pathology seems logical as an area for further consideration in the diabetic male, especially with the recent work of Faerman et al.[12] who found histological evidence of autonomic neuropathy in the neural fibers of the corpora cavernosa.

Since there is no known effective therapy for such sexual dysfunction, it is most important that the physician be certain that he is not dealing with impotence due to correctible causes. Assessment of drug therapy to watch for erective difficulties arising from the use of tranquilizers, antidepressants, antihypertensives or estrogens will be rewarded with an occasionally simple solution to what might otherwise appear to be a complex problem. Alcohol consumption, statistically, is a frequent factor in the appearance of impotence.

The differential diagnosis of impotence in the diabetic male revolves around other organic causes and the psychogenic etiology including the aging male variant described by Masters and Johnson.[13] A useful analysis of this differential is shown in Table 3 along the lines of presentation by Cooper.[14] Characteristically, diabetic men with organic impotence have continued sexual interest despite the slow onset of erectile dysfunction, often described as "50 per cent firm." They generally have an inability to masturbate or stimulate erection in any way.

The organically impotent male due to other causes such as impotence following prostatectomy usually has much more abrupt onset of impotence and a complete lack of ability to obtain morning erections or masturbate. Psychogenic impotence is generally abrupt in onset; libido is low and masturbation ability is maintained. A change of partner often alleviates the disorder. This variation of impotence is frequently reversible.[8] Depression and anxiety often accompany organic impotence, leading to a psychologic overlay.

The low percentage of impotence due to psychologic causes in this series of patients was most likely due to the nature of the patient population; the subjects came for medical treatment of diabetes on a regular basis, as contrasted with patients who seek a specialist, like a urologist, for a specific sexual problem. In most physicians' experience, strong psychologic concerns are more often the main factor in the latter group.

A study of sexual dysfunction in diabetes would be incomplete without mention of the importance of appropriate counseling for both spouses in such instances. The physician, although unable to offer a cure for the disorder can often alleviate a tense home situation by adequate explanation. This allows for misinformation and cultural bias to be corrected and provides an opportunity for each spouse to attain a greater degree of comfort in living with a difficult problem.

REFERENCES

1. Rundles, R. W.: Diabetic neuropathy. Medicine 24: 111–60, 1945.
2. Rubin, A., and Babbott, D.: Impotence and diabetes mellitus. J.A.M.A. 168:498–500, 1958.
3. Schoffling, K., Federlin, K., Ditschuneit, H., and Pfeiffer, E. F.: Disorders of sexual function in male diabetics. Diabetes 12:519–27, 1963.
4. Ellenberg, M., and Weber, H.: Retrograde ejaculation in diabetic neuropathy. Ann. Intern. Med. 65:1237–46, 1966.
5. Ellenberg, M.: Impotence in Diabetics: The Neurologic Factor. Ann. Intern. Med. 75:213–19, 1971.
6. Kolodny, R.C.: Sexual dysfunction in diabetic females. Diabetes 20:557–59, 1971.
7. Masters, W. H., and Johnson, V. E.: Human Sexual Inadequacy. Boston, Little Brown & Company, 1970.
8. Mayes, D., and Nugent, C. A.: Determination of plasma testosterone by the use of competitive protein binding. J. Clin. Endocrinol. Metab. 28:1169–76, 1968.
9. Croxton, F. E.: Elementary Statistics with Applications in Medicine and the Biological Sciences. New York, Dover Publications, 1959.
10. Rivarola, M. A., Faerman, I., and Jadzinsky, M.: Plasma testosterone levels in diabetic men with and without normal sexual potency. Excerpta Medica I.C.S., V. 38, 1970. (Abstracts of papers presented at the Seventh Congress of the International Diabetes Federation, Buenos Aires, Argentina, August 23–28, 1970.)
11. Weiss, H. D.: The physiology of human penile erection. Ann. Intern. Med. 76:793–99, 1972.
12. Faerman, I., Glocer, L., Fox, D., Jadzinsky, M. N., and Rapaport, M.: Impotence and diabetes. Excerpta Medica-Eighth Congress of the International Diabetes Federation, Brussels, Belgium. July 15–20, 1973.
13. Masters & Johnson, op. cit., chapter 12, p. 326.
14. Cooper, A. J.: Diagnosis and management of "endocrine impotence." Br. Med. J. 2:34–36, 1972.

AUTHOR'S COMMENTARY

Further analysis of the results shows the following: 48 per cent impotent and 8 per cent of the impotent group clearly had psychological presentations; 7 per cent improved with treatment of grossly uncontrolled diabetes; 33 per cent remaining largely "organic" in presentation.

When this study was completed, the office visit status of the randomly seen patients did not allow a detailed neurological examination.

Despite this fact, the group designated as impotent had about twice the incidence of neuropathy as the nonimpotent group. Conceivably, with motor nerve conduction and EMG studies, the differentiation would be greater.

The lack of difference that duration and mode of therapy made in the outcome of our group of patients can invite several interpretations. Certainly, many of the organically labeled group could be involved psychologically, providing a so-called "mixed" clinical presentation. This would lower to some extent the one-third incidence in the average diabetic male population that is included in this study. Most estimates of organic impotence in nondiabetic samples are at the 5 per cent level. The author is impressed with the high sexual interest found in the diabetic male with this complaint compared to the low libido found in the classically depressed male with sexual dysfunction.

The sleep research plethysmograph monitor device developed by Karacan et al.[1] and available commercially,[2] should help to clarify further the mixed clinical situations where the diabetic male has a suggestion of both organic and psychologic presentations. The diagnostic device should clarify the history of morning erections that can be difficult to elicit in many middle-age males. The presence of this function is very important in the sexual assessment, because many men conclude that lack of spontaneous erections to formerly erotic stimuli signifies definite impotence, when this tendency really relates more to the normal aging response as described by Masters and Johnson.[3] The presence of unconscious erections during sleep underscores normal neurological and circulating function as mentioned in the paper.

The lack of correlation with duration of diabetes should discourage the physician, since many professionals formerly have felt "the longer the duration of diabetes, the more inevitable the complication of impotence." This is *incorrect* reasoning which has added as much to the problem as the objective evidence contained in this study. Furthermore, to reason from duration of diabetes to need for prosthesis can promote unnecessary surgery.

The use of insulin, diet alone or oral hypoglycemic agents made little difference in the incidence of organic impotence. Many diagnosticians routinely test the G.T.T., since it appears to be the only significant laboratory test that is easily available to clarify the medical diagnosis.

In the later study by Schoffling, a few patients were included who acquired diabetes in the growth years (i.e., the juvenile diabetic patient). Many young men read in the lay press information derived in part from the references in this study and tend to extrapolate to their own subgroup. Physicians should discourage this tendency until more work is done on this particular subgroup of youth-onset diabetic patients. This author has not been impressed with men in the twenty-to-forty age group who have had diabetes for about ten to thirty years and who experience an increased amount of impotence. There are exceptions to this statement, including those young people who have neuropathy in the form of bladder paresis and foot deformities. Autonomic dysfunction that includes a potency problem would be expected with these clinical associations.

D.M.B.

REFERENCES

1. Karacan, I. et al. Sleep-related penile tumescence as a function of age. Am. J. Psychol., 1975, p. 132.
2. American Medical Systems, 3312 Gorham Ave., Minneapolis, MN 55426.
3. Masters, W. H. and Johnson, V. E. Human Sexual Inadequacy. Boston, Little Brown & Co., 1970, Chapter 12.

9

Sexual Function
in Hemodialysis Patients

NORMAN B. LEVY, M.D.

Since 1961 hemodialysis has been established as a feasible procedure by which patients with end-stage kidney disease can be kept alive indefinitely. Those who would have died of uremia are now able to live in a compromised but—in many instances—satisfactory life.

Prior to 1970, knowledge about the sexual dysfunctions of hemodialysis patients was restricted to case vignettes, usually involved exclusively with the issue of impotence of male patients. In 1972 Scribner estimated that about one-third of the men on hemodialysis are totally impotent, one-third partially impotent and one-third not impotent at all.[1] Despite the need for information about these problems, there were no systematic studies on the sexual dysfunctions of hemodialysis patients until recently.

Friedman and his associates attempted to obtain information concerning the interest in and actual experience of sexual intercourse from 13 married patients and their spouses.[2] Of the six wives responding, all reported that their husbands had no difficulty maintaining erections during sexual intercourse. However, in comparing their partners' current performance to the time prior to their illness, five stated that there was a marked decrease in the frequency of intercourse. Of interest is the fact that three of these five husbands reported the frequency of sexual intercourse as the same or just slightly less than that prior to symptomatic kidney disease.

In a study by Foster and his colleagues on 21 patients undergoing maintenance hemodialysis over a two-year period, three patients reported that they were never impotent, three that they were rarely impotent, three that they were occasionally impotent, two frequently impotent and ten always impotent.[3]

Abram and his associates conducted semi-structured interviews with 32 married male hemodialysis and transplant patients in a Veterans Administration hospital.[4] They also conducted interviews with 11 of the wives of these patients. Nineteen of these patients had functioning renal homografts at the time of the study, thus allowing a comparison of sexual activity prior to the onset of kidney disease, while on hemodialysis and after transplantation. The major indicator of sexual activity in this study was the frequency of intercourse. In this study "reduced potency" was defined as a decrease in frequency of sexual intercourse of 50 per cent or more (irrespective of cause) when compared to sexual activity prior to the onset of kidney disease. Seven patients had no significant decrease in sexual relations after the onset of disease or after the institution of dialysis. Fourteen patients reported reduced potency after the onset of renal disease and the remaining 11 patients had no significant decrease in sexual activity after the disease onset but reduced potency after beginning dialysis. The average frequency of sexual intercourse per month of the patients studied was 10.4 before the onset of uremia, 5.7 after the onset of uremia and before hemodialysis, and 4.0 while maintained by hemodialysis.

The most definitive and certainly the largest study to date has been performed by Levy who investigated the sexual adjustment of 429 adult hemodialysis patients by the use of a questionnaire.[5] Because he wanted patients to directly receive the questionnaire in the privacy of their homes, he enlisted the cooperation of the National Association of Patients on Hemodialysis and Transplantation (NAPHT), a national patient-consumer organization. They were the only possessor of a large number of names and addresses of these patients who comprise the majority of its membership. The questionnaire requested that all adult patients, defined as 18 years or older, answer all applicable questions. The establishment of the restriction to adults was necessary in order to gain the cooperation of this organization.

The questionnaire addressed itself to sexual functioning as measured by frequency of sexual intercourse in members of both sexes, prevalence of impotence in men and frequency of orgasm during intercourse in women. Patients were compared as to three periods of time: before the onset of symptomatic kidney disease (uremia), after being uremic but before the use of hemodialysis, and since being on maintenance hemodialysis.

Of the 1166 questionnaires mailed, 778 (67 per cent) were answered and returned; 536 respondents were patients, the others were interested professionals, laymen and relatives of patients. Of the 536 patients, 429 were on maintenance hemodialysis and 56 were transplant recipients. The majority of the patients, 78 per cent, were married; 16 per cent were single; 1 per cent were widowed; 3 per cent were divorced; 2 per cent were separated and the marital status of 1 per cent was not given. The ethnic backgrounds of the respondents were 91 per cent white; 6 per cent black, 1 per cent oriental, 1 per cent of a variety of racial backgrounds and 1 per cent failed to answer this question. The primary occupations of the patients prior to developing uremia were: 24 per cent skilled workers; 17 per cent professionals (8 of whom were physicians), 16 per cent housewives, 10 per cent sales people, 9 per cent students, 8 per cent business executives, 7 per cent managers, 4 per cent unskilled workers, 4 per cent in categories which could not be classified and 1 per cent did not answer this question.

Table 1. *Frequency per week of intercourse of men on hemodialysis*

	Never	Once or Less	Twice	Three or More	No Answer
Before Uremia	27	129	85	38	8
On Hemodialysis	135	114	16	4	18

As seen in Table 1, although 27 male patients never had sexual intercourse before uremia, 135 or five times that number never have sexual intercourse after being on hemodialysis. At the other extreme of frequency, 38 men had sexual intercourse three or more times per week prior to uremia. However, since being on hemodialysis less than one-ninth or four patients have intercourse that frequently. As seen in Table 2, the frequency of sexual intercourse of female patients showed a change in the same direction. Before the onset of kidney disease, 13 women never had intercourse but since being on hemodialysis, more than three times that number (47) never have intercourse. At the frequency of three or more times weekly, the numbers were 21 before being uremic, and only 8 after being on hemodialysis.

Table 2. *Frequency per week of sexual intercourse of women on hemodialysis*

	Never	Once or Less	Twice	Three or More	No Answer
Before Uremia	13	58	43	21	7
On Hemodialysis	47	62	15	8	10

Concerning the prevalence of impotence, patients were rated concerning whether or not they were partially or totally impotent. We defined impotence in this study as the inability to get or maintain an erection for sexual intercourse or decreased sexual desire to such an extent that the patient himself reported it as a problem. Total impotence was defined as total inability to have or maintain an erection for intercourse; impotence of a lesser degree was termed "partial." As seen in Table 3, 160 or 59 per cent of all men on hemodialysis considered themselves to be either partially or totally impotent.

Table 3. *Impotence in hemodialysis patients*

Partial	Total	Not Sure	No Problem	No Answer
95	65	23	89	15

Table 4 shows the frequency of orgasm in women patients during sexual intercourse. In hemodialysis patients, as seen in the two extremes of frequency—"usual" and "never"—there was a marked decrease in frequency of orgasm during intercourse since being on hemodialysis as compared to that prior to uremia.

Table 4. *Frequency of orgasm during intercourse of women on hemodialysis*

	Usually	Unusually	Never	Not Sure	No Answer
Before Uremia	90	14	12	10	16
On Hemodialysis	47	16	34	12	33

The data clearly indicate that patients on hemodialysis have major deterioration in sexual functioning. The men, however, seem to be more affected than the women.

Concerning the onset of sexual dysfunctions, approximately one-half of the men and one-third of the women found that the problems in sexual functioning emerged or worsened as they progressively became uremic, prior to starting hemodialysis. However, after hemodialysis only 24 (8%) of the men and nine (6%) of the women had some improvement in sexual functioning, whereas 100 (35%) men and 35 (25%) of the women experienced decline in sexual functions. This is a particularly paradoxic response since the use of hemodialysis is associated with improvement in all other physical functions. However, a large group of patients experienced worsening of sexual functioning. These data replicate with a larger number of patients—Abram's group of 32 patients in which the frequency of sexual intercourse was found to diminish as patients went on hemodialysis.[4] Kaplan De-Nour has made the general observation that the majority of problems of impotence occur after male patients are on maintenance hemodialysis programs and not before that time.[6]

ETIOLOGY

The cause of the sexual dysfunctions of hemodialysis patients must be physical as well as psychological. Physically, these patients are chronically and severely anemic and intermittently uremic. They suffer from the many problems to which their underlying illness and its treatment makes them prone. These include problems of bone dysfunctions connected with secondary and tertiary hyperparathyroidism. Their fistulae and/or shunts make them prone to circulatory and local problems connected with clottings and occlusions of these vessels. Several investigators have noted specific hormonal abnormalities in uremic patients.[7-9] Although the women have changes in menses, there are no specific hormonal variations reported in them. Among men, loss of testicular size and diminished sperm production seem to be related to depressed testosterone production. The data related to testicular, hypothalamic and pituitary interreactions are conflicting but suggest both a primary testicular defect as well as a problem in the normal feedback response of the hypothalamus. Some patients have combinations of depressed testosterone with normal luteinizing hormone levels or high luteinizing hormone levels and normal testosterone levels. Gynecomastia does occur in uremic males. It is usually bilateral, with occasionally tender breasts, but it is not associated with galactorrhea. Gynecomastia is not related to elevated estrogen levels, prolactin, luteinizing hormone, follicular stimulating hormone or increased estrogen-to-testosterone ratio.

Recent investigation in the biochemistry of sexual dysfunctions of patients with end-stage renal disease has indicated that parathyroid hormone and zinc seem to have some causal role. In a pilot study of seven male patients maintained by hemodialysis, Massry and co-workers treated them with 1,25-dihydroxy-vitamin D_3 to produce suppression of the parathyroid gland activity.[10] Psychiatric and hormonal evaluations were performed before and repeated two months after this treatment. Of the four of these seven patients who had been impotent prior to treatment, two experienced virtual resolution of the impotence, while one other potent patient also experienced increase in frequency of sexual intercourse.

Eight impotent hemodialyzed men were studied by a group of investigators at Georgetown University as to plasma zinc levels, sexual functions, testosterone, follicle-stimulating hormone and luteinizing hormonal levels.[11] All eight were partially or totally impotent and all had low plasma zinc levels. An experimental group of four of these patients had zinc chloride added to their dialysis bath; the other four served as a control group and had no change in their dialysate. The mean baseline plasma zinc level for the entire group was well below normal. One week after the addition of zinc chloride to the dialysis bath, plasma zinc rose to slightly above normal in all of the experimental group. Three patients in the experimental group reported "striking improvement" in potency two weeks after the addition of the zinc, while the other patients reported improvement after four weeks of therapy. In none of these patients did sexual function return to its predialysis level. The control group was unchanged. Of the four patients receiving zinc therapy, two had normal and two had low plasma testosterone levels. Following therapy, the low testosterone levels in the latter two patients rose to normal.

Both of the above studies are pilot rather than definitive investigations. They are small sample-sized, report behavioral data based on self-observation of subjects within a short span of time, and therefore lack an objective longitudinal overview. Both are studies of male patients only. However, like studies of tryptophan loss and the use of bromocryptine in the treatment of impotence, they require further investigation in broader samples. At this point there are some clues, but no definitive answers to the biochemical cause of sexual dysfunctions in these patients.

As to physiological causes, the data in the study by Levy, in which patients showed worsening of sexual functions as they went from untreated uremia to treatment with hemodialysis, may be explained on a psychological basis.[5] Hemodialysis may be perceived by men as being emasculating because of its association with the reversal of family role, and the passivity and dependency associated with this procedure. Sexual functioning in the male and urination are closely allied mentally because they are allied physically; both involve the penis. Thus, cessation in urination in men tends to be seen as emasculating, especially in men whose masculine identity is tenuous. In women, loss of attractiveness, menses and availability to engage in women-related activities may be seen as defeminizing.

Depression, which is the most common psychological problem of patients on hemodialysis, is associated with sexual dysfunction. A patient who is depressed usually has a diminished interest in sexual activity, or a continuing interest with diminished ability to perform sexually. A combination of physical and psychological factors may work synergistically. Thus, a patient whose sexual dysfunction may have a hormonal basis may perceive such dysfunction as a great blow to his sense of maleness or to her femininity and respond to this psychologically by further impairment in sexual functioning.

TREATMENT.

When physical factors are dominant, their treatment may be necessary in order for the patient to regain his sexual interest and/or ability.

Much can be done to combat the psychological effects of illness upon
these patients. Virtually all hemodialysis patients are unprepared for
the sexual complications of their therapy. Many assume that with the
initiation of hemodialysis and subsequent improvement of all other
physical functioning, sexual functioning will also improve. When there
is failure to improve sexually or worsening of sexual functioning after
being on hemodialysis, most patients confronted with the paradox respond with surprise. Some feel unique or "different" in some way
because they have a sexual problem. Among the most reassuring statements that can be made to patients is that they are not alone in this
problem, i.e., that the problem is commonplace. Prophylactically, it is
best that patients be prepared for the possibility of having sexual dysfunctions even before starting hemodialysis. Then, should sexual dysfunction occur, they will not tend to view it as peculiar to them but as a
complication of their treatment, and thus more readily call it to the attention of the treating physicians.

In differentiating physical as opposed to psychological impotence, the
presence of morning erections and erections for the purpose of masturbation favor a psychological cause. Dream laboratory tests may also be
helpful in making the differential. Stage 1 REM sleep is characteristically associated with erections in the male throughout his lifetime.
The ability of a patient to get an erection can be established by identifying this phase while asleep and measuring change in penis size. Thus,
should the patient be able to get an erection in Stage 1 REM sleep and
be impotent for sexual intercourse, it would argue in favor of a diagnosis of psychologically caused impotence. However, there may be a
mixed picture of both organic and psychological causes.

Many psychological syndromes, but especially depression and anxiety reactions, diminish sexual interest and/or ability. Early identification of these illnesses is essential because they may be treated either
by supportive psychotherapy or by the use of medication. However, as
a group, patients being maintained by hemodialysis tend to be rather
resistive toward psychotherapy.[12] This is due to the fact that denial of
illness—including psychological illness—is common among them[13]; as a
group they tend to feel they have had enough medical care, and they are
rather resistant to measures increasing their medical attention. As to the
use of medication, the two rules in the pharmacology of end-stage renal
disease are that the medicine given not be excreted by the kidney and
that it not be dialyzable. The former is necessary in order to avoid toxic
levels and the latter in order to avoid subtherapeutic levels. This rule

106

essentially eliminates the minor tranquilizers and lithium carbonate in the psychopharmacological treatment of these patients. However, phenothiazines—that is, the major tranquilizers such as chlorpromazine—may be used to treat anxiety, and the tricyclic antidepressants such as imipramine (Tofranil) and amitriptyline (Elavil) may be used in the treatment of their depression.

More recently, behavioral techniques such as those described by Masters and Johnson are being used in selective groups of hemodialysis patients with sexual dysfunctions. Although there are only a few workers in this field and only one published report to date,[14] these techniques do hold promise.

REFERENCES

1. Scribner, B.H. Panel In Living or Dying: Adaptation to Hemodialysis (N.B. Levy, Ed.) Springfield, Charles C Thomas, 1974, p.25.
2. Friedman, E.A., Goodwin, N.J. and Chaudhry, L. Psychosocial adjustment of family to maintenance hemodialysis-Part II. N.Y. State J. Med. 70:767, 1970.
3. Foster, F.G., Cohn, G.L. and McKegney, F.P. Psychobiologic factors and individual survival on chronic renal hemodialysis: a two year follow-up: part I. Psychosomat. Med. 35:64, 1973.
4. Abram, H.S., Hester, L.R. et al. Sexual functioning in patients with chronic renal failure. J. Ment. Dis. 160:220, 1975.
5. Levy, N.B. Sexual adjustment to maintenance hemodialysis and renal transplantation: national survey by questionnaire. Trans. Amer. Soc. Artif. Ind. Organs 19:138, 1973.
6. Kaplan De-Nour, A. Some notes on the psychological significance of urination. J. Nerv. Ment. Dis. 148:615-623, 1969.
7. Gupta, D. and Bondschu, H.D. Testosterone and its binding in plasma of male subjects with chronic renal failure. Clin. Chim. Acta 36:479, 1972.
8. Chen, J.C., Vidt, D.G. et al. Pituitary-leydig cell function in uremic males. J. Clin. Endocr. 31:14, 1970.
9. Lim, V.S. and Fang, V.S. Gonadal dysfunction in uremic men. Amer. J. Med. 58:655, 1975.
10. Massry, S.G., Goldstein, D.A. et al. Impotence in patients with uremia: a possible parathyroid hormone. Nephron 19:306, 1977.
11. Antoniou, L., Shalhoub, R.J. et al. Reversal of uremic impotence by zinc. Lancet 2:895, 1977.
12. Levy, N.B. Psychological studies on hemodialysis patients at the Downstate Medical Center. Med. Clin. N. Amer. 61:759, 1977.
13. Reichsman, F. and Levy, N.B. Problems in adaptation to maintenance hemodialysis: a four-year study of 25 patients. Arch. Intern. Med. 130:859, 1972.
14. McKevitt, P. Treating sexual dysfunction in dialysis and transplantation patients. Health Soc. Work 1:133-157, 1976.

10

Sexuality and Heart Disease

FRANCIS G. MACKEY, M.D.

Until very recently, little had been known or written about the subject of sexuality and heart disease. The answers given in response to patients' questions to their doctors about when and if they could resume sexual activity following a heart attack tended to be vague and often evasive.

Recent changes toward more openness in discussing matters pertaining to sex have resulted in more questions being asked of physicians. At the same time, knowledge is accumulating through research utilizing modern methods of cardiac evaluation, so that patients may now be given more assurance through considerably more precise answers to their questions.

Over the past five years, an inhospital cardiac rehabilitation program has been in operation at St. Jude Hospital and Rehabilitation Center in Fullerton, California. As a result of this program, we have become aware of the value of a combination of early physical reconditioning and an extensive effort to provide information to patients through a program of patient and family education.

During this period, we have searched the literature and accumulated experience mostly in the area of sexuality and arteriosclerotic heart disease, so our discussion in this chapter will be restricted to this area.

A PRECISE PRESCRIPTION FOR SEXUAL ACTIVITY

Currently there is growing medical interest in obtaining sound physiological facts for sexual counseling of cardiac patients. Rather than giving vague advice about when it is considered feasible to resume sexual activity, it is possible to develop a prescription for physical activity of all kinds including sexual activity. It is based upon a) knowledge of the energy requirements for sexual intercourse; b) application of the treadmill or bicycle ergometer stress test; and c) actual monitoring of the ECG during sexual intercourse by means of a Holter Monitor. Studies that have already been recorded in these areas will be reviewed.

First, let us review the physiological responses during sexual intercourse. The four phases are:

1. Excitement, erotic arousal.
2. Plateau—associated with foreplay and intromission.
3. Orgasm.
4. Resolution.

Maximal heart rates occur during orgasm.[1] These include transient tachycardia, hypertension and hyperventilation. Pulse rate, blood pressure and breathing increase progressively during erotic arousal and at intromission, attaining a maximum at ejaculation and orgasm, followed by an equally marked decline. Resolution takes place within one to two minutes. The duration of the maximum rate is brief, less than a minute.[2]

The magnitude of these responses (pulse rate up to 170 and respiration rates up to 30-60) have previously been reported in young healthy persons and have given physicians cause for alarm and undue caution in considering allowing cardiac patients to expose themselves to these levels of cardiopulmonary stress responses.

More recently, Hellerstein and Friedman[2] have studied cardiopulmonary responses in middle-aged, middle-class, convalescent persons with arteriosclerotic heart disease (ASHD) engaging in sexual activities with their wives of twenty or more years in the privacy of their bedrooms. The mean maximal heart rate during sexual activity corresponding to orgasm and ejaculation was 117 (range 90-144). The heart rate of the period encompassing the maximal heart rate, two minutes before and two minutes afterward, averaged 98.

This gives us a new perspective, indicating that most persons with ASHD and not in congestive failure can look forward to engaging in sexual activities with reasonable safety. It now becomes a matter of exploring the means by which relating precise testing measures may be employed to give patients specific rather than vague counseling.

THE EXERCISE STRESS TEST

It is important to recall that the stress test is used for two basic purposes: To diagnose the presence or absence of ASHD by assessing cardiac response while performing measured amounts of exercise and to develop a prescription for physical activity. It is the latter that will be discussed at this point.

There are a variety of protocols used to determine prescriptions for physical activity, but they are based on similar assumptions. Studies were done monitoring heart rate, ECG, blood pressure, and measurement of actual oxygen uptake with the Douglas bag. The double products, heart rate plus systolic blood pressure, were found to correlate with oxygen consumption, so the cumbersome system of measuring oxygen consumption can be eliminated.

The exercise prescription is developed by assessing the cardiac response during the exercise stress test and recommending that exercise be limited to the amount that causes the heart rate to reach approximately 75 to 85 per cent of this level. Rates higher than this can be hazardous, and rates less than this are thought not to produce conditioning effects. The upper levels are the ones to consider in counseling persons concerning their sexual activity.

There is no uniform agreement as to how long after myocardial infarction or coronary artery bypass surgery this test can be performed. In general, 4 to 6 weeks are recommended following surgery and approximately 6 weeks following myocardial infarction.[3]

A convenient way of determining oxygen consumption, estimated by measuring heart rate response, is in terms of mets. One met is the energy expenditure per kilogram of body weight per minute of an average individual sitting quietly in a chair or lying at rest. This amounts to 240 cc/min. In normal men, the mets increase twelve times at maximal exercise over those at rest. The heart rate correlates with the number of mets. On the average, middle-aged men who have recovered from an uncomplicated myocardial infarction have a maximum capacity of eight to nine mets.

Maximal activity during coitus approximates five mets for less than thirty seconds. During pre and post-orgasmic periods, the energy cost is about 3.7 mets. Bearing this in mind, one can establish the potential functional capacity by one's ability to perform activities of known energy cost or objectively on the treadmill or bicycle ergometer. If the cardiac patient can walk on a treadmill at three or four miles per hour asymptomatically and without undue elevation of blood pressure or ECG changes, his exercise capacity is five or six mets and equal to the energy demands of sexual intercourse and most jobs.

THE "SEXERCISE TOLERANCE TEST"[2]

Having developed a prescription for activity through the standardized stress test, one can counsel a patient regarding the timing and feasibility of resuming sexual intercourse following a myocardial infarct or heart surgery. At that time, an even more precise stress test may be employed. Hellerstein calls this the "Sexercise Tolerance Test": an ECG electromagnetic tape recording which monitors sexual activity in the privacy of the individual's home. One such device is the Holter Monitor, which can be worn for 24 to 48 hours. A diary is kept by the person being tested so that the ECG and heart rate response can be analyzed retrospectively in order to give more precise counseling to cardiac patients concerning their sexual activity.

POSITIONS DURING SEXUAL ACTIVITY

The assumption has been made that certain positions tend to reduce physical stress during sexual intercourse. The usual recommendation has been that the cardiac patient assume the passive role by being in the bottom position. Griffith[4] made the suggestion that the passive person sit on a low chair, head at rest on a cushion, feet resting on the floor. The active, healthy partner is above, on top of the sitting patient. However, Newman and Mansfield reached this conclusion through their research:

> Alternation in sex technique, such as using the man on the bottom position incurs no particular energy-saving advantage for male coronary patients. Blood pressure and heart rates have been directly measured and have been found to be the same in the man on top and the man on the bottom positions.[5]

They did not study the effects using the side-to-side position.

The results of this investigation should be a source of comfort for those who might find it an added emotional or physical strain to assume positions that to them might be strange and undesirable. Finally, it is a happy, loving, sexual experience that brings peace and contentment.

SEX WITH WHOM AND WHERE?

The often quoted study by Ueno,[6] a Japanese pathologist, indicated that an overwhelming majority of deaths among cardiacs occurred in men who were having clandestine sexual affairs with women in hotel rooms. This has led to the recommendation that male cardiac patients be advised to restrict their sexual encounters to their customary partners in the privacy of their own bedrooms. It is reasonable to assume that adultery can be hazardous to health if combined with fear and guilt or the excessive use of drugs and alcohol to loosen inhibitions.

On the other hand, Scheimann[7] says that hostility, frustration, and boredom can conceivably do harm, while the right kind of release with the right partner can be rejuvenating and life-enhancing.

There are indeed two sides to the coin. It is wise, therefore, to find out if there have been serious marital problems affecting sexual relations prior to the development of heart disease. Seeking solutions to these problems as part of the total assessment and treatment of the patient is needed in addition to the purely physical evaluations noted above.

OTHER HAZARDS

1. *Extremes of temperature*—whether very cold or very hot (especially with high humidity). The heart has to work much harder just to maintain normal body temperature. The room in which sex takes place should be at a comfortable temperature.

2. *Exercise and eating*—Digestion makes its own demands on the heart and one should wait at least three hours after eating a heavy meal before having sex.

3. *Excessive alcohol*—While alcohol tends to loosen inhibitions, if taken in large amounts it can be harmful. A recent study[8] indicated that as little as two cocktails can measurably reduce the cardiac output in persons who have a damaged heart. It is commonly thought that alcohol relieves the discomfort of angina by improving coronary circulation. On the contrary, alcohol dilates the superficial vessels producing skin flushing, and reduces coronary circulation. Alcohol, like barbiturates, Librium, Valium, Equanil, and others is a sedative—hypnotic drug. It has a depressive effect and can have a striking inhibitory effect on libido. This can result in increased requirements of physical energy to accomplish a satisfactory sexual experience.

4. *Fatigue*—Sexual functioning when one is fatigued is impaired under normal circumstances. Fatigue that accompanies diminished cardiac function can be readily compounded, so the times for sexual encounters should be selected when one is well rested.

PHYSICAL CONDITIONING AND SEXUAL PERFORMANCE

Hellerstein and Friedman's[2] investigations showed that sexual activity among persons with ASHD was influenced favorably by enhancement of fitness through systematic physical training. Initially, 21 per cent of ASHD subjects experienced angina pectoris or its equivalent most commonly during the resolution phase of sexual activity. After participating in a physical conditioning program, 30 per cent of the ASHD patients (and 39 per cent of the initially symptomatic subjects) experienced an increase in frequency, and 40 per cent an improvement in the quality of sexual activity. The frequency and severity of symptoms decreased in 67 per cent of ASHD subjects who initially developed symptoms during sexual activity.

Stein[9] conducted similar studies and demonstrated that the peak coital heart rate, and by implication, coital myocardial oxygen requirements, decline as the post-myocardial patient attains improved levels of fitness consequent to interval exercise training.

In the patient limited during coitus by anginal pain or other manifestations of ischemia, such as a decrease in the peak coital heart rates may be associated with a decrease in symptoms and consequent improvement in sexual functioning.

REHABILITATION EFFECTS:

1. Although rather minimal in conjugal lovemaking, physiologic costs of sexual activity to the cardiac patient can be lessened by an exercise training program. The improvement in performance capacity, lessening of catecholamine output, and sensitivity after training may have a beneficial carry-over into sexual activities.[10]

2. Exercise training may help sexual performance; however, the converse is generally untrue. Sexual activity cannot be substituted for the more traditional training programs because, although it may incur heart rates of 70-85% of maximum, that rate lasts only 10-30 seconds. To be an adequate training stimulus, sexual activity would have to sustain the training heart rate for 20-30 minutes three times a week.[11]

POST-SURGERY—SPECIAL PROBLEMS

The patient who has had bypass graft surgery is a candidate for early ambulation and rehabilitation care. Following recovery from the surgical procedure, an exercise test would help to identify any residual ischemia or myocardial inadequacy. If performance capacity is poor and ischemic ECG manifestations are severe, the graft should be suspected. If full activity has been achieved and no ischemic ECG changes are present on exercise testing, graft patency is probable and the patient can be encouraged to enter a training program to achieve and maintain optimal functional capacity. The patient who has had post-ventricular aneurysm resection is similar to the patient with a healed myocardial infarction.

Patients with inadequate pumping function may benefit from ju-
dicious training programs which enable the fixed cardiac output to be
used with maximum efficiency by reducing heart rate and improving
oxygen extraction by the peripheral tissues. These patients may be
good prospects for training because non-infarcted muscle is usually
well-perfused and the mechanical problems of too much scar tissue or
not enough chamber may well be improved by the enhanced function
of the remaining well-perfused, viable muscle.[12]

HYPERTENSION AND SEXUAL ACTIVITY

Hypertension is commonly associated with arteriosclerotic heart disease and questions often arise in this area. Concerning patients with
hypertension alone, Fries states:

> Sexual intercourse is not dangerous in patients with con-
> trolled hypertension. Although it is well known that blood pres-
> sure rises severely during the sex act, there is no documented
> evidence that this will precipitate cerebral vascular accidents.[13]

EFFECTS OF HYPERTENSIVE MEDICATIONS ON SEXUAL FUNCTION

The problems that occur with hypertension most often relate to the
effects of the drugs taken to control the hypertension. Probably the
most common effect of the rauwolfia drugs is depression of libido and
even impotency.

RETROGRADE EJACULATION

Sympathetic nerves control a sphincter muscle at the vesicourethral
junction which closes during ejaculation. In male patients taking guanethidine (Ismelin), this sphincter fails to close and there is retrograde
ejaculation into the urinary bladder. Patients who are given guanethidine should be told of this possibility so that they will not be alarmed in
case they develop orgasms without emission.[13]

Another effect is that produced by ganglionic blocking agents that interfere with potency and delay or inhibit ejaculation. In the order of
likelihood of producing this effect are:

Pentolinium (Ansolysen)
Mecamylamine (Inversine)
Guanethidine (Ismelin)
Methyldopa (Aldomet)

Drugs which rarely, if ever, have adverse effects are:
Oral Diuretics
Hydralazine (Apresoline)
Propranolol (Inderal)

Gifford, prominent authority in hypertensive disease at the Cleveland Clinic, states:

> In my opinion, the combination of an oral diuretic, hydrala-
> zine, (Apresoline) and Propranolol is one of the most effective
> regimens for the control of hypertension, mild or severe, and
> is the least likely to cause impotence or to inhibit ejaculation.[14]

Specific measures to provide protection from hypertensive complications include the following:

1. A supervised program of conditioning exercises to allow for greater exertional tolerance, and to achieve lower blood pressure. Several studies suggest that cardiovascular mortality rates vary inversely with previous physical conditioning.

2. Prophylaxis with nitrates (glyceryl trinitrate, amyl nitrate) which lowers systolic pressures 10 to 30 mm. Hg within 10 minutes and may last from 5 to 30 minutes. Side reactions of headache due to dilatation of small meningeal vessels and nitrate syncope due to a secondary vagal response occur in a certain percentage of patients.

3. Timing of the medication to assure maximum effectiveness in controlling the blood pressure during the time sexual activity is expected (parenthetically, the more potent drugs likely to be used in hypertension may cause impotence or inhibited ejaculation for the male).

4. Elevating the head of the bed 10 to 14 degrees to reduce maximum pressure effects of recumbency.

5. A period of rest after coitus is advisable to avoid sudden orthostatic drop in blood pressure upon standing.

6. Include the spouse for discussions of the entire matter, enlisting support in sexual matters and avoiding damaging misconceptions.[15]

MEDICATIONS THAT MAY HELP

Nitroglycerin taken before sexual intercourse may prevent angina pectoris in persons anticipating having it. Propranolol may also be effective in preventing the symptoms of angina through its beta blocking effect on the sympathetic nerves. Caution is in order, however; as Howard[15] reminds us, this drug blocks the cardiac responses necessary during exercise by limiting heart rate and cardiac output. During maximum levels of exercise, the ventricular myocardium requires simple tachycardia, sympathetic limitations, and increased contractibility in order to meet oxygen requirements. Propranolol, by reducing the heart rate, left ventricular minute work, and cardiac index, enhances the development of left ventricular failure during exercise stress. Propranolol should not be used in a patient with borderline congestive heart failure.

ADVICE TO PATIENTS REGARDING WARNING SIGNS

1. Chest pains during and after sex.
2. Heart palpitations that continue for a quarter-hour or more afterward.
3. Breathlessness that continues a quarter of an hour or more afterward.
4. Sleeplessness apparently caused by the exertion of sex.
5. A "knocked out" feeling the day following sexual activity.[16]

PSYCHOLOGICAL CONSIDERATIONS

Up to this point, the discussion has dealt with physiological considerations. A myocardial infarction and/or cardiac surgery obviously has an impact on the patient's psyche. This warrants our careful attention.

Anxiety is the first reaction encountered in the intensive cardiac care area. It is managed in the acute phase with appropriate medications such as: Valium, Librium, or barbiturates (sedative-hypnotics). This is coupled with firm and optimistic reassurance and a limited explanation of the nature of the disease and what is happening at the moment. This tends to allay anxiety.

Denial is almost always an initial response and can be regarded as a desirable early psychologically protective mechanism. It usually evolves gradually into a state of reactive depression. It is this state, if deep and unduly prolonged, which may interfere with a return to satisfactory sexual functioning. Hackett, evaluating the psychological aspects of patients with myocardial infarction at Massachusetts General Hospital, observed that heart patients usually go into varying degrees of depression about the third day in a coronary care unit. This is about the time patients begin to realize that they won't die and then begin to think about their future, their jobs, and their family life.

Such depression is associated with insomnia, a feeling of hopelessness, sadness, tearfulness and self-despair. The depression usually lasts about three months. During this time, other manifestations that become evident are diminished energy, loss of interest in usual activities, including sexual intercourse. Hackett and most others agree that antidepressant drugs are not useful in this kind of depression. Instead, we should concentrate on dispelling the myths surrounding heart attacks.

Bowden[17] at Texas Health Science Center in Dallas believes that it is a mistake to treat patients immediately with antidepressants or refer them to a psychiatrist. This does not give persons the opportunity to cope successfully with their depression on a more independent level.

At this point, anger may intervene. Men in particular find the demonstration of anger more appropriate and acceptable behavior than the show of tears. It is important that staff members recognize this as an expected reaction and not directed to them personally, so that they do not respond to anger with anger but with kind, understanding and positive types of action.

It is my belief, and I find others agreeing with it, that depression, if not inappropriately prolonged or profound to the point of becoming suicidal, can be a positive and creative experience. It can be a time of long hours of quiet withdrawal, introspection, self-awareness and assessment into which one may retreat, perhaps for the first time, from the senseless whirl of the intensely competitive work-a-day world. A beginning can be made to reach out and explore ways to significantly change life-style to reduce or eliminate previously existing risk factors such as: heavy smoking, dietary indiscretions, uncontrolled alcoholic intake, and disregard for the management of hypertension. A new openness to changing sex role stereotypes may be generated. One may find it a welcome relief to be able to abandon the former "macho" attitude of regarding sex as a performance and begin to approach sexuality as a tender, loving, creative experience.

SOCIAL AND VOCATIONAL

Although 80 per cent of patients with myocardial infarctions are able to return to work within three months—most of them in their former jobs—some find it necessary to modify their vocations and in some instances opt for early retirement. Many employers, not appreciating the potential for continuing employment, harshly terminate these people or divert them into unimportant positions. This can have a potentially devastating effect in terms of self-worth, or may impose temporary or permanent role-reversal. It can have a serious impact on the individual's self-image and in turn, on his sexual relationships. Skilled psychological, social and vocational counseling becomes extremely important under these circumstances.

Myron Brenton in his book *Sex and Your Heart* states:

> It seems fair to conclude that cardiac patients, surgical and non-surgical alike, just aren't getting the care for their psyches they're getting for their bodies. Oh yes, if the patient really goes into an intractable mental funk— becomes paralyzed with fear, suicidal, or otherwise goes off the deep neurotic end—there's likely to be a psychiatric referral.

> But if he seems to be carrying on somehow at home, at work, and in the community; if he doesn't articulate his troubles; if he holds back about a drastic curtailment of his sex life, then no matter how stressful his circumstances may be, it's very problematical whether he'll get the effective help he needs.

> Why? Resistance to psychiatry and resistance to the team approach are two important reasons. At the present time in American medicine the team approach, especially when a member of the team would turn out to be somebody from the psychological community, isn't a very promising situation. Many of the surgeons' queries for the book felt that, insofar as surgery is concerned, the surgeon should be at the center of the state, providing the patient with support and reassurance. Many of the internists and cardiologists queried felt they were psychologically hep enough and well enough acquainted with their cardiac patients to be their source of strength and guidance. Bringing in somebody else, these specialists felt, would only serve to dilute the central doctor-patient relationship.

> If this were the best of all possible worlds, every physician who treats the physical ailments of mankind would be plentifully endowed with the temperament, training, and time needed to offer supportive psychotherapy as well. Unfortunately, it isn't and they aren't.[18]

Specifically, what does the heart patient need to help him cope with his or her illness? Dr. Duane Rumbaugh, Professor of Psychology at San Diego State College, who has done much work in the field of cardiac rehabilitation, lists the following patient needs:

1. Education about his impairment.
2. Knowledgeable persons with whom he can feel free to express his fears, discuss his apprehensions, and to ask about the most intimate questions he has.

118

3. Encouragement to communicate with people in the face of his tendency to withdraw.
4. Having his interests cultivated or born anew.[19]

Myron Brenton concludes as follows:

> Given the epidemic character of heart disease in the United States, maybe what's needed is a radically different approach to rehabilitation, one that doesn't rely in piecemeal attempts at restoring the patient to health physically and psychologically. Maybe what's needed in those communities whose cardiac populations warrant it is a blockbuster assault on the various manifestations of the disability—community cardiac rehabilitation centers.[20]

Since Brenton made this statement in the first edition of his book in 1968, we in 1972, and an increasing number of other hospitals have experienced the value of this kind of care for the cardiac patient. In our project, a team of physicians, nurse specialists, physical and occupational therapists, psychologists, social workers, and an exercise physiologist have worked closely together as an interdisciplinary team of health professionals to treat the whole person with complex physical and social problems.

In response to Rumbaugh's statement of the cardiac patient's number one need (education about his impairment), we are in the process of developing a series of color cassette video tapes dealing with the problems of sexuality in heart disease. It will be shown to patients and their families in groups or on closed circuit TV in the patient's hospital room. Much of the information presented in this chapter has been transferred into language that is understandable to the average non-professional person for use in such presentations.

Fear, ignorance and misinformation prevent many people with mild to moderate cardiovascular dysfunction from enjoying sexual relations. Yet sex is one of the essential human needs, and we believe it can be more fully enjoyed by a great majority of persons with heart disease if professionals and non-professionals can take advantage of the increasing number of cardiac rehabilitation programs becoming available throughout the country.

REFERENCES

1. Masters, W.H. and Johnson, V. Human Sexuality. Boston, Little Brown, 1966.
2. Hellerstein, H. and Friedman, E.H. Med. Aspects Hum. Sexuality, Mar., 1969.
3. Elliott, R.S. and Miles, R. Consultant, p. 23, Sept., 1973.
4. Griffith, G. Med. Aspects Hum. Sexuality, Oct., 1973.

5. Newman, E. and Mansfield, L. Scientific Sessions for Nurses (Abstr.). American Heart Assn., Dallas, Tex., Nov. 19, 1974.
6. Ueno, M. Sex and Your Heart. New York, Award Books, 1968, pp. 25-26.
7. Scheimann, E. Sex Can Save Your Heart and Life. New York, Crown Publishers, 1970, p. 218.
8. Gould, L., Reddy, R. and Goswani, K. Chest 63:943-947, 1973.
9. Stein, R. Circulation 55 (5), May, 1977.
10. Exercise Committee, American Heart Association.
11. Heart Disease and Sex: Responses to Questions. Med. Aspects Hum. Sexuality 5:24, 1971.
12. *Ibid.* 11., p. 33.
13. Fries, E. Med. Aspects Hum. Sexuality, Oct., 1973.
14. Gifford, R. Med. Aspects Hum. Sexuality, Oct., 1973.
15. Howard, E.J. Med. Aspects Hum. Sexuality, pp. 89-90, Oct., 1973.
16. Brenton, M. Sex and Your Heart. New York, Award Books, 1968, p. 60.
17. Bowden, C. Presentation. Southern Med. Associates, Review.
18. Brenton, M. *Op. cit.,* pp. 165-166.
19. Rumbaugh, D. Sex and Your Heart. New York, Award Books, 1968, pp. 168-169.
20. Brenton, M. *Op. cit.,* p. 171.

11

Stroke and Sex

DOMEENA C. RENSHAW, M.B., Ch.B., M.D.

Victims of stroke have been called the "half dead" in oriental culture, a graphic statement illustrating that most persons who survive have a residual hemiplegia. The dreaded disease is unwelcome, unpredictable, and often crippling. *Stroke* is indeed an emotional word, conjuring up visual images of wheelchairs, walkers, catheters, canes, splints, speech problems, and drooling facial paralysis. Nearly all survivors are confronted by chronic disability.

Modern medicine can investigate and diagnose, rehabilitate and mobilize, but as yet we offer dim hope for cure or reversal of the pathology already caused by cerebrovascular accidents. Prevention of stroke is still a future eldorado, since the complex hemodynamics of raised blood pressure, weakened vessels and clotting mechanisms that contribute to its cause are poorly understood and therefore, still unpredictable. Today's antihypertensive drugs vary in the effectiveness with which they produce a sustained and steady reduction of blood pressure.[1] Good medical management of hypertension hopefully prevents the complication of stroke, which is always a high risk in severe hypertension.

HYPERTENSION AND SEXUAL ACTIVITY

There is a range from zero to 10 in what internists tell their hypertensive patients about future sexual activity[2,3] and of sexual effects of antihypertensive medications.[4] One physician said: "I tell them to watch it with sex." This is just enough for patients to avoid sex altogether or to develop impotence. Anxious self-watching is not conducive to relaxed, natural sexual functioning. It is the rare physician who regularly and carefully asks patients about sexual function on each follow-up visit. Bowel and urinary functions, yes, but not about sex. An explicit sexual history is unfortunately a clinical rarity because sex is a sensitive subject. "Why embarrass the patient?" is a much used alibi to cover the doctor's own discomfort with explicit sexual questioning.

During the first 72 hours, a stroke is usually an overwhelming body reaction and is life-threatening. A sexual history is irrelevant during this period. In the first recovery days, questions about sexual functioning are not high priority for the patient, physician, or spouse. However, sex questions become important and imperative to discuss for the patient and spouse (as a couple) before the time of the hospital discharge. A prominent internist when asked recently about sexual problems in stroke victims, said openly: "I've never asked. I don't know. The only ones who ask me about sex are the hypertensives."

On leaving the hospital, a stroke patient may have much anxiety. The body has been damaged, the brain has been damaged, and the sense of self may also in some persons be severely shaken by changes in motility, vision, speech, etc. Life-saving equipment and medical personnel are being left at the hospital. This may be a frightening thought. Now the patient must face spouse and family without outside aid. The mirror may cause deeply saddened feelings at the decline in appearance and movement. Loss of strength may be followed by possible loss of job as a real threat. The patient may also fear losing love, even more so if there was marital discord before the stroke. Going home means the possibility of trying out what is now left of self-function. There will be much uncertainty about all previous skills, particularly about sexual skills. The patient may be embarrassed to try sexual relations with a disability such as limb paralysis when there now exists a real risk of rejection due to appearance or of fumbling or failing. The physician may have been vague or may have avoided mentioning that sexual activity may safely resume as soon as the couple desires. A history of previously good sexual functioning is, of course, diagnostically and predictively important.

TAKING THE SEXUAL HISTORY

When attempting to obtain an in-depth sexual post-stroke history, it is worth remembering that some persons have a sense of self-blame and guilt when they become sick. In Western culture sex has been a leading cause of guilt. Therefore, patients may state that the stroke was punishment for "sexual sins." Sometimes they anxiously carry on internal bargaining with God, promising to avoid sex completely if survival occurs.

Readjustment for such patients takes understanding and careful discussion with the physician to resolve such possible but needless guilt by giving accurate medical education regarding the cause, unpredictability and clinical course of the illness.

Often patients may wish they had died at the time of the cerebrovascular accident: "Then I would not have to drag this ugly body and twisted face around," said one bitter woman, whose previously low self-esteem was now totally shattered by the catastrophe she was unable to face alone. Another 39-year-old attractive woman with residual hemiplegia was sexually rejected by her husband who had an affair, stating "I hate sickness and now I have an invalid in my bed." They came to Loyola Sex Clinic about his lack of sexual desire for her, dating from the day of her ruptured cerebral aneurysm.

The literature offers few well-documented clinical studies of post-stroke sexual function. Ford and Orfirer in 1967 reported on 105 stroke patients under 60 years of age: 60 per cent said their sexual appetite was the same or greater; 43 per cent had decreased frequency of coitus; 22 per cent had increased coitus; and 35 per cent gave incomplete information.[5] Most of the 105 stroke patients reported the same subjective sexual desire as previously but lessened opportunity to satisfy their desire due to the partner's fear or abhorrence. However, this attitude may also reflect the patient's own feeling about self rather than the partner's. This needs explicit discussion with both partners present so that assumptions may be avoided.

A clearer understanding of sexual dysfunction becomes possible and more lucid if the patient and physician have knowledge of normal sexual responses. Sexuality starts physically in utero and continues developmentally into our adult male or female identity. Psychic and social stimuli are important and are mediated through all of the special senses—olfactory, optic, auditory, gustatory—as well as through general touch sensation. All of these may sexually stimulate or inhibit. Genital sensory tactile stimuli may similarly enhance or restrict sexual responses which may be either reflexive (clothing) or deliberate (love play). Interoceptive reflex sexual responses are known to arouse or inhibit through bowel or bladder stimuli.[6] Orgasm is a natural, total body response, involving intact brain, spine, nerves, muscles, blood vessels, heart, lungs, and genital organs.

Unless the cerebral insult is very severe, the sexual response, both anatomically and physiologically (presumably mediated through the limbic system and spinal cord) is usually spared. The neurophysiology and neurochemistry of the human sexual response are, at our present stage of knowledge, still mostly theoretical. Research exists from both primate laboratories and postneurosurgery patients[7,8] which is just beginning to add to the now well-known mechanical knowledge of normal male and female sexual responses and dysfunctions.[9,10]

NEUROLOGICAL FACTORS

Autonomic. Possible sexual dysfunctions resulting from stroke depend on the extent of the cerebral damage. Partial erections, impotence, ejaculation, and decreased lubrication in the female are all theoretically possible if there has been damage to higher centers of the autonomic nervous system. These are unusual occurrences in survivors of stroke.

Sensory. The commonest outcome of stroke is left hemiplegia. For sex counseling of the hemiplegic and partner, it is important for the physician to know that in addition to motor weakness there may also be absence of or excessive sensation on the entire affected body side ("numb" or "dead" may be the patient's description). Visual changes (homonomous hemianopsia) accompanying left hemiplegia will prevent recognition of a person or objects in the range of the left outer and right inner semicircle of the visual field. In the give and take of sexual overtures and subsequently during actual coitus, it would be helpful for the physician to suggest that the healthy partner approach the patient from the intact visual field; also that he or she use stimulating touch on the intact body half and ask the patient to give verbal feedback regarding which side of the bed he or she would prefer for optimal sexual agility.

Motor. Muscle weakness and unstable joints on the paralyzed body side will produce mechanical difficulties and awkwardness until the couple works out practical common sense ways of overcoming these problems. A handle on the headboard, a higher footboard, a trapeze, pillows or simply alternative coital positions might be suggested. Loss of sphincter control might be assisted by manually emptying the bladder before sex. Each patient usually develops his or her own ways to cope as privately as possible with such an embarrassing disability. Soiling is undoubtedly contraerotic. The physician should encourage open discussion that this may occur. To assist problems in this area a Pamper beneath the supine patient helps and is easily disposable.

Speech loss of lesser or greater severity may occur with stroke. This may also vary with emotions. It then becomes important for the couple to use nonverbal cues and be helped to develop and to recognize such a code. One wife rushed in distress to her neurologist when her now aphasic husband blurted out a four-letter word. He had high desire and expressive paralysis. But under his stress, the obscenity emerged. The very sensitive neurologist smiled and reassured the surprised wife and explained that all her husband was asking for was to restore their sex exchange. It is a tremendous boost to the patient's self-esteem to remain sexually desirable and be approached by the partner. This wife was able and happy to do so. Such exchanges should be encouraged, if there is mutual desire.

Emotional factors. If the patient fears performance or another stroke, or if anger between the couple exists, sexual problems will inevitably arise and the couple should be so informed. Both anxiety and anger block relaxed sexual arousal.

Timing for general mobilization of a stroke patient is of the essence— the earlier the better, within limits of physical tolerance. The same thing is essential for sexual mobilization—the sooner the better for the patient's self-esteem and recovery.

Expected and quite normal reactions to a stroke may include demoralization of both patient and spouse: crying; anger; anxiety; agitation; loss of sleep; initial and temporary denial "must be a mistake—perhaps we should go to Mayo's for a check-up..." Time should be set aside for talking in private with the aware physician to answer questions about the stroke and thus assist in coping and adaptation. Realistically, the demoralization assists in the adaptation to life at a lesser level of action. Stoic endurance or resignation with personal courage and expressed religious faith may relieve doctor and family alike, and many such cases of quiet heroism and respondent family devotion are seen in the everyday care of persons with chronic illness.

There are times, though, when an already tenuous marital equilibrium is shattered by further disability. Divorce or abandonment without divorce of a stroke patient by a distressed spouse is not unknown. A clinical depression may occur, with or without agitation or suicidal feelings or attempts. Characteristically in a clinical depression, all of the appetites are lowered: for food; for sleep (causing irritability, tiredness and further anxiety); for sex (further stressing an already anxious spouse or the depressed patient who may worry that the sexual changes—loss of interest, impotence, anorgasmia—are due to the stroke when in fact they are due to the depression);[11] for life itself (a sense of hopelessness and helplessness may lead to suicidal preoccupation, planning attempts). Hypnotics may be stored and tragically used.

Such pathologic reactions must be seriously regarded by all physicians entrusted with the care of stroke patients, since suicide is the mortality of depression. Suicidal risk should be carefully evaluated by open questions: "Have you thought about dying? What kind of thoughts? Have you thought of harming yourself? How? Have you been bothered by thoughts of suicide? How have you handled these? Has anyone in your family made suicide attempts? Have you? How? Did you talk to anyone about it? Would you consider talking to someone about it?" This is an essential lead-in to a needed psychiatric consultation, since hospital care may be critical to avoid catastrophe. Talking about suicide does not cause it, but it may prevent it. Stroke victims in their middle years are as prone to involutional agitated depressions as others and as excellently responsive to a course of electroshock therapy. Collaborative management requires close working together of internist, anesthetist and psychiatrist.

The non-suicidal, clinically depressed stroke patient of any age may be managed by any physician with or without backup psychiatric consultation. Adequate dosage of antidepressants from 100 to 300 mg. tricyclic, examples: Sinequan (doxepin) is the least cardiotoxic; Elavil (amitryptyline); Tofranil (imipramine) is today preferably used as a single bedtime dose to obviate the use of hypnotics or daytime drowsiness. For elderly apathetic stroke patients who are unable to tolerate antidepressants due to glaucoma or for other medical reasons, a trial with Ritalin (methylphenidate) 5 to 10 mg. daily at 8:00 a.m. may make a positive difference in the quality of their day. It can improve their alertness, activity, hygiene and eating, prevent excess daytime dozing and restore a night-time sleep and sex cycle, the latter probably due to their improved responsiveness.[12,13] When the clinical depression responds, the reported loss of sexual desire, impotence, or anorgasmia will totally reverse.

Chemical factors. Alcohol used in excess is perhaps the most common cause of the first episode of secondary impotence.[14] Alcoholics have a high incidence of sexual problems, and stroke is not a cure for alcoholism! A good sexual history should always include details of alcohol intake. Many needed and life-sustaining drugs cause impotence as an autonomic side effect, the most common being psychotropic drugs widely used for emotional problems.[15] Major and minor tranquilizers, some antidepressants, antihypertensives, and antihistamines are all likely to be used by the stroke patient and should be checked in the history. It should also be remembered that stroke in young patients may be caused by intravenous drug abuse. Such patients may continue their habit post-stroke, and this possibility should be questioned and rehabilitation attempted.

Factors of aging: Together with their peers, stroke patients age and deserve to learn the expectable and normal sexual changes lest they think these due to stroke and develop needless anxiety-related interference with sexual performance. For all women over 50 years, there will be thinning of the walls of the vagina and reduced lubrication, responsive to local hormonal cream, replacement lubrication in the form of KY jelly or saliva for comfortable coitus. For *all* men over 50 years, there will be partial erections due to normal changes of elasticity of connective tissue and of blood vessels. With prolonged petting and loveplay partial erections may improve, but the angle of the full-erect penis to the abdomen will not be as acute as formerly, yet this should not impede penetration nor orgasmic pleasure unless sexual ignorance causes anxiety. Ejaculations may occur before full erection. The point of ejaculatory release will be less clear, the amount and force of the ejaculate will be lessened. For both sexes the objective intensity of the increased heart rate, respiratory rate, muscle tension with sexual arous-al and climax will somewhat lessen, but subjective sexual desire and enjoyment remain the same and often increase. Also for both sexes, the frequency of intercourse may decrease, but this is highly individual and also is related to *previous* frequency of coitus. The more active the per-son has been, the more active the person remains even into late life. This is equally applicable to the stroke patient.

SEXUAL THERAPY AND COUNSELING

All of the foregoing is basic sex education which may in certain cases be sufficient to reverse a sex problem such as sexual avoidance when this is due to sexual ignorance, now corrected by the physician-authority. A conservative reading list may reinforce the gains.[16,17] So may a few explicitly illustrated booklets shown to a couple together (to avoid mis-interpretation that the physician has prurient motives) before their ap-pointment so they may present their questions to the doctor.[18] A tape recording about sex and stroke in the doctor's voice may similarly be utilized for a couple to listen to together before an appointment. A fol-low-up visit in 3 or 4 weeks can check the progress.

If basic sex education alone has been insufficient, the physician may make a contract for 5 visits spaced once a week with the couple for brief sex therapy which will take one hour each, and the fee should reflect this designation of time and recognition of their problem. As a sex educator, the respected physician-authority can provide knowledge of the body and how it does or does not work by being as explanatory for the genitals as for the pancreas in the physical and sexological ex-aminations. In the presence of patient and committed partner, the physical state is explained (for example: heart, lungs, abdomen, blood vessels and nerves are all fine. The blood pressure is borderline, but salt-free diet and loss of 5 pounds should take care of that. I'll check again next month"–) Then the *sexological examination* is done, ex-plaining to both: "Here are the testes in the scrotum. The left normally hangs lower (some men worry that they are deformed). Feel it (partner's thumb and index finger). Here is the vas which carries the sperm. Feel it. The penis is uncircumcised and of normal size. This whole general area, including the buttocks and anus, is very erotic in both sexes. Here is where the squeeze technique can be applied to enhance the duration of erections. Feel it (always suggest this—some women are fearful or inhibited about touching the penis).[11] The physician's guidance is most beneficial. For the woman's sexological examination a similar approach is used, plus a mirror so that she may see her genitals clearly (in lithotomy with the head of the table elevated 45 degrees). "Here are the outer lips, the inner lips, the clitoris is here under my index finger. Mary put your index finger over mine while I take mine away. Do you feel the clitoris? Roll it side-to-side. Good. John, put your index finger on Mary's which she'll take away. Do you feel the clitoris? Roll it side-to-side. Good. The clitoris has only one function, sexual arousal, so unless it is directly or indirectly stimulated, arousal may be more difficult. Like John's, this whole general area and buttocks are potentially sexual. This is the vaginal opening. The lining is shiny and moist. This is normal secretion (or has a slight infection or could use some special cream—). Just relax and breathe out slowly. Keep your mouth open and breathe out. Relax, good. Now I'm doing a pelvic. Everything's fine. Now contract very tightly around my fingers with the vaginal muscle. Tighter. Good. It's a circular muscle like around the eyes and mouth, and you can contract it at will and practice it to enhance sexual pleasure for both of you. Now breathe out again, relax. There, that's the speculum in. Now let's adjust the light and mirror so you can both see the cervix. Can you see it? Now I'll take a quick Pap smear and we're all done."

This sex education is the physician's special domain; it may not be delegated and cannot be overestimated in its therapeutic value. For many, it obliterates the sexual ignorance of a lifetime. And it does more. It gives, usually for the first time, *permission* from a respected authority to look at, know, touch, understand the sexual self (and at home to enjoy it). This bonds the couple together and to the physician. The sexological examination is not easy for the couple. The more comfortable the physician, the more comfortable the couple will be. The first few times this new modality is practiced by the physician, there may predictably be normal physician discomfort. However, with skill, practice and positive results, will come increasing comfort for the practitioner.

Open discussions of early sex inhibitions, misconceptions, and relationship problems begin and continue from the first visit onwards. The sex disability may be impotence or anorgasmia or loss of interest or dyspareunia or vaginismus. Very often it predates the stroke, but it merits treatment whenever help is sought. With the couple present, the doctor suggests daily home exercises of relaxation and sensual enjoyment, mutual total body massage for 30 minutes daily, no matter what the symptoms.[16] Also coitus in the first two weeks is de-emphasized and forbidden. Thus, immediately for both partners, performance anxiety and fear of failure are alleviated. The man is encouraged to be receptive and relaxed and overcome his feelings of being threatened by sexual initiative and activity in his partner. The woman is told to relax and enjoy her pleasure in her turn, but to be imaginative, sexual and sensitive when approaching him. Both learn that acceptance of various pleasurable erotic stimuli results in erections, arousal and lubrication that come, go and return. Such success is self-reinforcing. *Time* and *testing* can then build self-confidence, which is the essential cure for each. Progress continues to more specific exercises for specific sexual symptoms.[16]

Early morning masturbation daily in a relaxed and lying-down position is suggested as a transient exercise for impotence and for anorgasmia in the first few weeks of treatment to restore function and confidence. Each partner is told to spend five minutes in private doing this, and is told to do so in the partner's presence so both may understand rather than resent. If the patient is able to accept the physician's encouragement and prescription to do this assignment, prognosis for restored functioning is usually good. Permission to use erotic fantasy should be given to an inhibited person. This distracts the couple from spectatoring themselves and getting anxious about failure to erect or climax. Suggest next that one time at least, a full masturbation be done in the other's presence. This is of great value in bringing masturbation out of the secrecy of the bathroom into the relationship as an intermediate step towards restored coitus. This is often difficult. It is a crisis of intimate sharing and is usually a turning point in therapy, for it is educative regarding the function and friction preferences (intensity/lightness) of the other during sexual expression.

Woman-on-top position is then suggested for quiet penile containment in the vagina. This is helpful for impotence, premature ejaculation, dyspareunia, vaginismus and also anorgasmia. Ten minutes daily for 3 days is spent on this. The wife is instructed to stuff the partially erect penis into the vagina as both of them continue general petting which usually results in an erection within the vagina. Coitus is then recommended with this valuable woman-on-top position. Each is again advised to use their favorite erotic fantasy to distract self from anxiously "spectatoring" their own performance. Success, often within 2 to 10 weeks, is between 40 to 80 per cent for co-operative couples with this non-complex technique of sex therapy. Those who do not respond may then be referred to a Sex Clinic for more intensive help.[19]

In summary, far too little is known scientifically of specific dysfunctions related to stroke. Some sexual difficulties relate to emotional causes: ongoing anxiety about a potential recurrent stroke; overwhelming fear after the catastrophic event; anxiety about sexual failure or performance; possible unresolved guilt; or a clinical depression. These are all reversible with either an explicit, clear discussion of sexual function or sex counseling or appropriate antidepressants from their internist or family physician (with both partners present). This may even make a profound change in the way the couple relates after the stroke. Separate loneliness can be avoided in the remaining years by promoting optimum closeness. The quality of life for the stroke survivor may thus be improved by the aware, humane physician.

REFERENCES

1. Prichard, B.N.C. Variations in the modification of cardiovascular responses by sympathetic inhibitor drugs. Proc. Roy. Soc. Med. 62:84, 1969.
2. Griffith, G.C. Sexuality and the cardiac patient. Heart Lung 2:70, 1973.
3. Lord, J.W., Jr. Peripheral vascular disorders and sexual function. Med. Aspects Hum. Sexuality 7:34, 1973.
4. Simpson, F.O. B-Adrenergic receptor blocking drugs in hypertension. Drugs 7:85, 1974.
5. Ford, A.B. and Orfirer, A.P. Sexual behavior and the chronically ill patient. Med. Aspects Hum. Sexuality 1:58, 1967.
6. Weiss, H.D. The physiology of human penile erection. Ann. Intern. Med. 76:703, 1972.
7. Bors, E. and Comarr, A.E. Neurological disturbances in sex dysfunction; 529 patients with spinal cord injury. Urol. Serv. 10:191, 1960.
8. Malin, J.M., Jr. Sex after urologic surgery. Med. Aspects Hum. Sexuality 7:245, 1973.
9. Masters, W.H. and Johnson, V.E. Human Sexual Response. Boston, Little Brown, 1966.
10. Masters, W.H. and Johnson, V.E. Human Sexual Inadequacy. Boston, Little Brown, 1970.
11. Renshaw, D.C. Sexual dysfunctions of depression. In Kiev, A. (Ed.) Somatic Manifestations of Depressive Disorders. Amsterdam, Excerpta Medica, 1974, p. 86.
12. Renshaw, D.C. Management of the elderly patient. Chicago Med. 76:229-233, 1973.
13. Kaplitz, S.E. Withdrawn, apathetic geriatric patients responsive to methylphenidate. J. Amer. Geriatric Soc. 23:271-276, 1975.
14. Renshaw, D.C. The sexual problems of alcoholics. Chicago Med., May 17, 1975.
15. Renshaw, D.C. Sex and drugs. Nursing Care 11:16-19, 1978.

16. Belleveau, F. and Richter, L. Understanding Human Sexual Inadequacy. New York, Bantam Books, 553-05959, 1970.
17. Our Bodies Ourselves—A Book by and for Women. New York, Simon and Schuster, 1977.
18. Yes Book of Sex, You Can Last Longer; Yes Book of Sex, Masturbation Techniques for Women. Multimedia, 1525 Franklin, San Francisco, Calif.
19. Koch, L. and Koch, J. Consumer guide to therapy for couples. Psychology Today 33-72, March, 1976.

12

Prostatectomy, Sexual Disabilities and Their Management

Saul Boyarsky, M.D., Rose Boyarsky, Ph.D.

INTRODUCTION

Prostatectomy is a common experience of older men in most Western countries. In the United States and Great Britain, it is estimated that as many as one in ten men will undergo a prostatectomy at some time in their lives.[11]

Many anxieties arise in relation to surgical procedures, and even more anxieties arise from a procedure on an organ involved in sexual and reproductive function.

The purpose of this chapter is to review what is known and to provide information and principles regarding the effect of prostatectomy on sexual function. We will discuss the various types of prostatectomy, the differential diagnosis of prostatic enlargement, the sexual consequences of prostatectomy, certain associated medical and iatrogenic disorders, and popular and nonurological misconceptions in the area. No attempt has been made to provide a thorough urologic discussion, since this is available in any standard textbook on urology or prostatectomy.

HISTORICAL ASPECTS

For the first third of the century, prostatectomy was performed either by the suprapubic route (the suprapubic prostatectomy) or by the perineal route (the perineal prostatectomy). There were two types of supra-

134

pubic prostatectomy—a one-stage and two-stage procedure. The two-stage procedure was really a preliminary suprapubic cystostomy to establish drainage for the bladder and kidneys so that the patient could recover enough strength and organ function to withstand the actual prostatectomy itself.

The prostate patient of those decades was usually very ill, often admitted in acute urinary retention, possibly with hemorrhage, suffering from hydronephrosis, uremia or serious urinary tract infection. There were no antibiotics and no blood banks; anesthesia was crude and hazardous by present-day standards. As a result, prostatic surgery was surgery of the last resort, with considerable mortality and morbidity.

In the 1940's and 1950's, there was remarkable progress in surgery, anesthesia, and medicine in general, and in urology in particular. Transurethral resection of the prostate, the endoscopic method, was perfected. This was followed by development of the retropubic prostatectomy.

The connotation of prostatectomy has changed greatly. At the turn of the century, it was an operation which carried a mortality of almost 40 per cent; it now carries a risk on the order of 1 per cent. In certain favorable groups of patients, the risk is well below 0.5 per cent mortality. Whereas the complication rate in pre-antibiotic days was 20 to 50 per cent, we now see many of our patients going home after one week of hospitalization with little significant discomfort, inconvenience or complications.

RECENT ADVANCES

At present, prostatectomy can be an elective procedure, just as is cataract surgery. The patient and the physician choose an operative time when it is apparent that the procedure will be necessary and inevitable, but before complications have set in. Diagnostic techniques have improved so that patients can be operated before they develop pathologic sequelae or other conditions which will lead to complications.

The enlightened physician, urologist and patient are very likely to view prostatic obstruction as a condition for continuing care and to choose the time of surgery electively.

New surgical and hospital techniques, antibiotics, blood transfusions, improved anesthetic techniques, and better catheters have spelled out progress which has changed the picture of prostatic surgery immensely. The infection rate, stricture rate, postoperative fevers and rigors, lost catheters and midnight alarms are in large part now preventable.

There still remain, however, patients who carry the fears and misconceptions of the past and who remember the pain, dread, prolonged hospitalization, and even death. They carry a fearful memory which is no longer realistic in present-day urology. As a result, some may deny their symptoms, postpone or avoid urological care on the basis of these mis-understandings and thus make happen exactly those complications they most fear.

In fact, the current safety of prostatectomy has allowed it to be ex-tended to many feeble, very old and very ill patients who never before were able to benefit from this surgery. Heretofore, these patients were condemned to living with a catheter for the remainder of their lives.

Today's patient walks into the hospital before he has developed any hemorrhage or urinary infection or after his infection has been con-trolled by antibiotics. Even if he has severe diabetes, hypertension, car-diac disease, a cardiac pacemaker or severe arteriosclerosis, he is an appropriate candidate for prostatic surgery because of the lowered risk. Should there be any difficulty during or after surgery, intensive care units, hemodialysis, pulmonary intensive care and other organ support systems are available to handle the crisis.

At this time, the greatest number of prostatectomies are performed by the transurethral route, up to 95 per cent in some centers. The rest are retropubic or suprapubic, depending upon the history of that medical center or urologist's experience. Very few prostatectomies are performed by the perineal route. One of the prime reasons for this is that in contrast to the other three types of prostatectomy, the perineal prostatectomy is believed to produce impotence in a high percentage of patients.

Because many patients strongly associate the prostate itself with sur-gery, benign prostatic hypertrophy must be distinguished from prosta-titis. Prostatitis is an inflammation or infection of the prostate. Although it is a disease of all ages, it is particularly predominant in the young. It is not a surgical disease, except in rare instances when resistance to ther-apy is associated with stones or extreme chronicity. But when it coexists with benign prostatic hypertrophy, it must be treated and controlled be-fore surgery is performed to minimize postoperative complications.

The young adult may suffer temporary prostatic obstruction from his prostatitis if the swelling is severe enough. But this rarely leads to sur-gery, although it may occasionally lead to temporary catheterization. The physician may do well to make sure the patient really understands the distinction between prostatic hypertrophy and prostatitis.

BENIGN PROSTATIC HYPERTROPHY AND CARCINOMA OF THE PROSTATE

In order to understand the salient features of prostatectomy, it is neces-sary to discuss the clinical entity of benign prostatic hypertrophy. Nodu-lar hyperplasia of the prostate or "BPH" is the most common neoplasm of

136

the prostate. The etiology of benign prostatic hypertrophy is still unknown but it accounts for some 80 to 90 per cent of prostatectomies performed. The other 10 per cent is largely due to cancer of the prostate.

While the inflammatory disease of prostatitis can occur at any age, most frequently in the young, the two neoplastic diseases show a frequency of distribution rising from the age of 40 to a peak in the sixties with incidence of cancer rising in each decade thereafter.

Carcinoma of the prostate can cause symptoms similar to BPH and is often difficult to differentiate from BPH. It may coexist with benign prostatic hypertrophy and thus a differential diagnosis may not be completely made until after surgery has been performed. The life-threatening concerns of having a carcinoma may be realistic on the part of the patient; they may be shared by the urologist. Both urologic surgeon and patient may need to await completion of a thorough preoperative work-up, performance of the surgery and the pathologist's examination of the excised tissue to make a positive differential diagnosis. Even a needle biopsy of the prostate used as a preoperative diagnostic test is not 100 per cent accurate.

Carcinoma of the prostate may be discovered during the preoperative studies for prostatectomy or it may be reported during the postoperative convalescence as a previous unsuspected finding in the tissue excised by the urologist. The symptoms of carcinoma of the prostate vary: they may simulate those of benign prostatic hypertrophy; the carcinoma may be asymptomatic and detected only by chance examination, or it may produce a full blown picture of prostatic obstruction with added symptoms of carcinoma—pain, anemia, weight loss and weakness.

Like most carcinomas, carcinoma of the prostate embodies a spectrum of severity ranging from a relatively benign course to an extremely malignant disease. Some carcinomas of the prostate are only histologically malignant, they show no tendency to metastasize. The patient with this type will usually die of something else before he dies of his carcinoma. Other carcinomas are highly malignant, metastasize widely and will kill the patient in a matter of months, no matter what therapy is given. Most carcinomas lie in between. Although carcinoma of the prostate is extremely common, it is not considered to be an outgrowth of benign prostatic hypertrophy but rather to co-exist with it. Both diseases are common in the same age group.

Carcinoma of the prostate is amenable to estrogenic or female hormone therapy, or to bilateral orchiectomy which removes the main source of androgenic hormone that sustains the growth of the prostate. The feminizing effects of the hormonal therapy for carcinoma of the prostate include the development of gynecomastia and occasionally hot flashes. Impotence frequently results.

Since about two-thirds of patients with carcinoma of the prostate have been estimated to respond to hormonal therapy, the patient often has the difficult choice of deciding whether he wants to extend his life or continue to enjoy his sexuality. Since total or radical prostatectomy and high-dose, high-voltage x-ray therapy also impair potency to a significant degree, the patient's alternatives for therapy add little to the probability of retaining sexual function. If the tumor is discovered early, the choice can be made to postpone therapy till the need is pressing and symptoms start to bother. However, Ellis and Grayhack report that almost half of men studied who were potent prior to hormonal therapy retained some degree of sexual activity afterward.[2]

Radical surgery is indicated only if clinical studies show the prostatic carcinoma to be at a low enough stage to be limited to the prostate and not to have spread beyond the confines of the gland itself. Otherwise, experience has shown that the tumor cannot be completely excised, and any hope of cure is unrealistic. Radiation therapy and hormonal therapy are very helpful against tumors which have spread beyond the gland, but the duration and extent of their benefit is not predictable.

Besides presenting the patient with possible impairment or abolition of his sexual activity, the diagnosis of carcinoma of the prostate elicits the emotional trauma of facing death, suffering, separation, and the curtailing of one's life and one's working capacity. These traumata produce anxieties and fears of their own which interfere with the patient's quality of life. His sexuality may be beset in more diverse and more severe ways than from the prostatectomy and loss of genital function alone. Stating it differently, libido as well as potentia may be threatened.

Radical surgical therapy for carcinoma of the prostate requires that the prostate be excised down to the level of the external sphincter of the membranous urethra and that the bladder be reanastomosed to this urethra. Although the technique has been perfected, a small number of patients will predictably have stress incontinence, and some 2 to 5 per cent of patients may be left with severe incontinence. This risk is considered necessary in order to remove the cancer completely. Those cases which are amenable to surgical care are identified by a thorough preoperative work-up which today includes the sophisticated tests of bone, liver and spleen scan and radioimmune acid phosphatase determinations.

It is particularly in the group of young patients who have undergone radical surgery for carcinoma of the prostate that the penile prosthesis has value.

DIAGNOSTIC TESTS

The clinical importance of the benign disease of prostatic enlargement is the degree of obstruction to the outflow of urine. If the prostate doesn't restrict urine flow, then no matter how large the prostate, it is not significant clinically. Younger or more vigorous patients who are active and have good bladder function may show surprisingly little obstructive effects in spite of impressive enlargement. They are not candidates for surgery. It is important to understand that the surgery is done for relief of *urinary* obstruction. To the extent of present-day knowledge, the enlarged prostate is still functioning well. The basic urologic study here is to determine the degree of bladder obstruction by the prostate via rectal examination, cystoscopy and radiographic procedures such as intravenous urograms or pyelograms and urodynamic tests.

Though manipulative or invasive, and although they may produce transitory discomfort, these diagnostic procedures have no lasting effect on sexual function and potency. Patients may need to be reassured of these facts so as to avoid unnecessary fear and anxiety or iatrogenic impotence.

ALTERNATIVES TO PROSTATECTOMY

Benign prostatic hypertrophy is still rightfully considered a condition requiring surgery even though there are medications and treatments which will improve the symptoms of prostatectomy somewhat. Obstruction caused by the prostate is usually partial and slow in developing. The bladder is capable of compensating so that the course of the disease is variable and intermittent. Estrogens, newer progestational hormones, antiestrogens and other drugs, such as candicidin, will cause regression in the obstruction and size of the prostate.

Bladder-stimulating drugs such as bethanecol have not been used successfully because of the acute nature of their effect. Recently another category of urethral and bladder neck-relaxing drugs in the form of sympatholytics, the alpha-adrenergic blocking agents, have shown promise.[1]

There is no "magic bullet" for this disease, however. Emptying the prostate gland of its secretions by massage or ejaculation can relieve the pressure of the hypertrophied gland on the urethral lumen. Such benefits, however, are temporary and partial. The prostate tissue is so elastic and resilient that the urethral lumen is compressed shut as the tissues spring back. Because of the progressive nature of this benign neoplastic growth, the bladder will eventually decompensate because the urethra becomes occluded. Theoretically, every patient, if he lives long enough, may need operative relief.

It is helpful for patients to recognize and avoid those types of events which will aggravate their symptoms or produce acute retention, such as the use of diuretics, drinking excessive amounts of fluids, the diuretic effect of liquor and beers, and the diuretic effect of exposure to cold for many hours at a time.

Patients can be taught to empty their bladder by slow voiding or double voiding (allow the urine to drain slowly and steadily, or making a second and even third attempt to empty the bladder) so as to reinforce the remaining functional capacity of a partially obstructed bladder and hence postpone the prostatectomy.

INDICATIONS FOR SURGERY

If a patient has his sleep interrupted more than three times nightly, or if he has serious difficulty in emptying his bladder; if his daily activity is disturbed by the impairments of urination or frequency; if the objective findings of abnormally high residual urine or impaired flow rate are present, then the obstruction has probably become severe enough to warrant surgical intervention. If certain complications or sequelae appear, such as uncontrolled or recurrent bleeding or infection, the development of bladder calculi, hydronephrosis, acute urinary retention or other complications such as diverticulum, then again, surgery may be indicated.

If the patient cannot empty his bladder at all, or if his bladder empties poorly (i.e., carries a large post-micturitional "residual urine") then an indwelling urethral catheter must be passed and left in place to drain the bladder until surgery can be performed.

The indications for prostatectomy are fairly clear in the urologist's mind. Although a precise formula cannot be given, the degree of obstruction, the residual urine in the bladder, the impairment of the urinary stream, the flow rate, the development of ureteral obstruction or hydronephrosis, the recurrence of infections, the possibility of an underlying cancer, the patient's reaction to his symptoms, the severity of symptoms, his disability, the availability of surgical care, are the factors to be taken into account.

PREPARING THE PATIENT

Patients approach the urologist and the possibility of such an operative procedure with a variety of emotions. They should be encouraged to ask and to talk about their concerns.

It is important to talk long enough and freely enough with patients so that any fears, misconceptions and unfounded beliefs which patients have regarding the effect of prostatectomy and prostatic disease upon their lives will surface. It is useful to inquire about their experiences, particularly about friends, acquaintances and relatives who have had similar diseases or procedures.

A brief explanation should be given of their diagnosis, the planned procedure and the consequences. One must ascertain whether there is confusion regarding diagnosis, type of procedure, possibility of consequences or complications, and the prognosticated outcome. Patient expectations of the results of the procedure and alleviation of symptoms must be realistic.

Legally, this explanation is necessary as part of "informed consent." Many urologists use diagrams, brochures and pamphlets, and some even use tape recordings or movies to ensure that the patient has at least heard about the procedure and its possible complications.

Other questions may lurk in the patient's mind and not be expressed. He may harbor questions such as:

Will I lose my sexual ability?

Will my partner leave me?

Will I regain my sexual abilities?

Does this mean I have cancer?

Will this restore my fertility?

Only by talking to patients in a non-prejudicial manner and by allowing them to voice their questions and concerns can one elicit the information needed to handle the emotional problems properly. These problems include (but are not limited to) the sexual.

It is not a narrow matter of avoiding lawsuits for mismanagement, but the larger one of obtaining adequate information so as to enhance the operative results, communicate clearly the expectations and restore the patient to adequate normal function—that is: to bring this man through his surgery well in all areas of his life. Our stated policy to all patients is that *there is no such thing as a "foolish question."*

THE SURGICAL EXPERIENCE

At this point it is necessary to explain in greater detail what is performed during prostatectomy. What is called a prostatectomy for benign disease is really a prostatic "adenectomy" or a partial excision of the diseased and expanded "core" of the prostate. Only for cancer or prostatitis with prostatic calculi, is a total prostatectomy performed.

The adenectomy is a removal of the substance of the prostate which has become hyperplastic and obstructed the prostatic urethra, thus interfering with the flow of urine from the bladder. The larger the gland, the more clearly delineated is the plane of separation between the compressed true residual prostate and the benign tumor, and the easier the dissection for removal.

The gross configuration of the benign tumor varies from patient to patient, often with some intrusion of the mass through the bladder neck back into the bladder. Occasionally, it dissects under the trigone of the bladder or even towards the sphincter along and down the urethra. At open surgery, retropubic, suprapubic or perineal, the adenoma is dissected out—in part under direct vision and in part by palpation. At transurethral resection, the adenoma is curetted out electrosurgically, piece by piece, taking care to preserve landmarks and vital structures. In all of the procedures, the surgical capsule of the prostate or the compressed true remaining prostate is preserved.

Transurethral resection is often viewed by the patient as "non-operative" since it is performed without abdominal incision and entirely through a resectoscope, a large cystoscope. Urologists appreciate the enhanced patient comfort, but must balance the surgical factors in their choice of procedure.

Depending upon the residual damage to the bladder neck from the ingrowth of the adenoma, the dilatation produced at surgery, or the actual resection of the bladder neck performed at surgery, the bladder neck can be left open so that the prostatic lumen or fossa communicates continuously with the bladder. Such a defect can be postoperatively detected radiologically in many patients.

The bladder neck is the site of the internal bladder sphincter, an organ which has a genital as well as urinary function under sympathetic nervous control. Normally it is closed during ejaculation so as to prevent the entry of semen into the bladder and also to facilitate its expulsion along the urethra. If this bladder sphincter mechanism is opened by the prostatectomy or by the disease, the semen is expelled into the bladder instead of through the urethra externally. This is the phenomenon of retrograde ejaculation.

Some patients (and occasionally their spouses) are disturbed by this. They require preoperative forewarning and postoperative reassurance. Younger patients who suffer from retrograde ejaculation for reasons which do not interfere with semen production, and who are concerned about fertility, can be helped to fertility by recovery of the semen from the bladder and instillation in the vagina by artificial insemination.

Frequently, men of the prostatic age have testicular atrophy and other conditions which cause infertility and azoospermia. Their spouses are rarely of a child-bearing age. As a result, fertility per se is rarely a real issue. The change in orgasmic feeling may, however, be an issue, especially if the man has not been prepared for this eventuality.

These considerations must enter into the preoperative discussions with the urologist.

POSTOPERATIVE INCONTINENCE

There is a low incidence of urinary incontinence after prostatic surgery; most of it is temporary and responds to medical therapy. This is a distressing complication for patient and surgeon alike. Proper informed consent includes discussion of the risk of incontinence.

Some patients are at high risk for post-prostatectomy incontinence. These patients must be warned of the higher risk and studied preoperatively so that special measures may be taken. Therapy for incontinence may include the use of a penile clamp or a urinary collection device. It is rarely necessary to re-operate to treat the urinary leakage.

THE URETHRAL CATHETER

A urethral catheter is frequently used during the preoperative and postoperative course of prostatectomy. Catheters are unpleasant and uncomfortable but need not be painful. The presence of the catheter in the urethra can induce an erection temporarily or repeatedly. The patient should be reassured that there is no lasting damage to his sexual abilities from the use of a catheter.

POSTOPERATIVE CONVALESCENCE

The postoperative course of recovery is not sudden, prompt, and final. It is gradual and occasionally interrupted. Patients may have all of the symptoms which brought them to the doctor: frequency, urgency, dysuria, incontinence accidents, and episodes of hematuria or acute retention. They may require rehospitalization, recatheterization, cystoscopy, passage of sounds or catheters for calibration, and antibacterial therapy. These setbacks usually clear rapidly and readily.

None of these postoperative discomforts would be expected to have any permanent effect on sexual function. Most urologists instruct patients to abstain sexually until their check-up four to six weeks postoperatively. This is to avoid complications, such as hemorrhage. Occasionally, one suspects that a patient's postoperative hemorrhage was induced by premature resumption of sexual activity. There is little or no documentation of the effect of sexual activity in the immediate postoperative stages, but there is no reason to doubt the clinical wisdom of proscribing sex until healing is complete.

POSTOPERATIVE MORTALITY

Between 1953 and 1965, mortality due to prostatectomy dropped to 2.1 per cent. It had been 8.5 per cent from 1942 to 1950.[16] A mortality rate of

1.3 per cent was reported by Melchior et al.[15] in 2223 consecutive trans-urethral resections of the prostate where the average age was 70 years. The 30 patients who died averaged 74.5 years of age. Cardiac problems accounted for half of these deaths. The authors of this report point out that actuarial tables showed that 4.8 per cent of American white men who are 70 years old die before they complete their 70th year. They suggest that this statistic be kept in mind when advising surgery. The complication rate for this group of patients was 17.3 per cent or 383 patients who had some form of non-fatal morbidity. It was the patients in poor general condition who showed a greater incidence of complications. There were 81.4 per cent who had no problem whatsoever.

SEXUALITY AND PROSTATIC SURGERY

Although there is extensive literature on prostatectomy and the mention of sexuality is interspersed throughout, it is only in the last two decades that much attention has been paid to the continuation of sexual function in these patients. This is due to the pioneering research of Kinsey (1948), Masters and Johnson (1965) and Finkle (1959, 1960).[3,4,9,14] The greater longevity of people, and the increase in the proportion of elderly in our population, along with other advances in geriatrics, has brought these problems to the fore.

Consonant with the historically changed picture of prostatic disease and surgery has been the emphasis in medicine and surgery on preserving the quality of life in addition to merely saving lives. This includes a greater attention to the effect of prostatectomy on sexuality.

There are no direct effects of benign prostatic hypertrophy itself upon potency, ejaculation or orgasm. The disease may interfere with sexual activity, however, by producing ill health or depression and through specific symptoms such as pain, infection, urinary frequency, nocturia, dribbling or enuresis. Interference with sexual function in prostatic disease may follow prostatic surgery; this may be due to the psychological interferences of fears, anxieties and expectations or to the cultural interferences of myths and misconceptions.

Erection depends on integration of afferent and efferent impulses in the sacral cord erection center and in the thoracolumbar cord. It requires an intact autonomic nerve supply to the penis and an adequate blood supply to its erectile tissue. Any interference with the nerve or blood supply can interfere with erection, ejaculation and orgasm.

Without going into detail about the physiology of erection and ejaculation, it is apparent that operative intervention anywhere along the regulatory nervous or circulatory pathways to the genital tract and penis may depress, interfere with or abolish sexual functioning.

   This occurs with abdominoperineal resection for removal of a rectal carcinoma, in Leriche's syndrome (which produces aortic occlusion and impairment of blood supply to the penis), or when pelvic or lumbar sympathectomies are performed.

   Impotence has also been reported following other surgical procedures such as abdominoperineal resection, abdominal aortic aneurysmectomy, aortal iliac endarterectomy, aorto-femoral bypass, abdominal aortic aneurysmectomy, dorsal or lumbar sympathectomy (particularly after bilateral resection of L-1 and L-2 ganglia), pelvic surgery near the hypogastric plexus, the pre-sacral plexus, the inferior mesenteric plexus, and operations on the lower bowel. Impotence has been reported after fracture of the pelvis and after high retroperitoneal lymphadenectomy.[8] The surgical approach for open perineal biopsy impairs potency, but less frequently or severely than for perineal prostatectomy. Impotence has also been reported after transurethral sphincterotomy which is performed from within the urethra, particularly if the incisions are made laterally at the 3 o'clock and 9 o'clock position. Perineal prostatectomy interferes with erections presumably because it, like the other surgical procedures, dissects the nervous pathways to the base of the penis. Prostatectomy turns out to be only one of many procedures which can jeopardize the nervous regulation of erection.

   It is necessary to separate the effect of specific dissection or trauma to the nerve supply of the penis from impotence due to a psychological problem, to a pre-existing impotence, or to impotence from loss of sexual interest or loss of sexual opportunity. The literature has not always been clear as to whether impotence following prostatectomy is temporary or permanent. There is also missing in the literature a report of the quality or degree of effort made to treat impotence in order to reverse it should the neurologic damage have been only temporary. More careful clinical observations are needed, and better neurologic observations postoperatively to determine what function has really been lost and what can be recovered. Adequate preoperative study is needed to find out if the disability existed beforehand or was merely reported postoperatively for the first time.

   The effect of prostatectomy on sexuality varies with the procedure performed. Of all the types of prostatectomy, only perineal prostatectomy, which is now the most infrequently performed, has produced impotence in roughly two-thirds of patients. Some of these patients remain potent. Suprapubic prostatectomy, retropubic prostatectomy and transurethral resection need not and do not threaten potency. In these procedures, if careful preoperative histories are taken and those patients who are impotent preoperatively are subtracted, the incidence of postoperative impotence is relatively unchanged. Studies show that certain patients do change categories after surgery; a certain number of patients regain their potency following these three types of prostatectomy, whereas other patients lose it. It is likely that factors other than the operative dissection itself have been responsible.

More radical surgery in which the entire prostate, seminal vesicles and base of the bladder are removed for carcinoma of the prostate produces impotence, even when performed by the retropubic route. It would appear that the extent of the dissection of the pelvis and disturbance of the nerves to the genital tract and the penis may be as important as the type of operation or disease. For example, Herr has reported that 20 of 32 patients averaging 61.2 years of age with prostatic cancer were sexually active and remained so at six months after pelvic lymphadenectomy and iodine-125 implantation.[8]

EJACULATION

When it comes to ejaculation, the effect of the various types of prostatectomy is more nearly uniform.

All types of prostatectomy, particularly the transurethral, interfere with ejaculation even when they may not have interfered with orgasm. A high incidence of retrograde ejaculation is reported by patients. There is some recovery over the passage of months or years. This is further evidence that erection and orgasm can and should proceed unimpaired even though ejaculation is lost.

In a study of ejaculatory functioning following prostatectomy, Windle and Roberts[19] found that 55 per cent of 90 patients lost the ability to ejaculate, but only 12 per cent or 10 patients became impotent. (The importance of considering the patient's sex life prior to operation was demonstrated. Of 119 patients undergoing prostatectomy, only 89 had normal sexual activity prior to surgery. Twenty-two patients had unsatisfactory function after surgery, eight due to distress over retrograde ejaculation and fourteen due to impotence. One patient made no attempt to have sexual activity.) In twenty of thirty patients with the ability to ejaculate postoperatively, only six were found to have spermatozoa in their semen specimens.

In a control group of patients who had intraperitoneal and inguinal-scrotal operations, five developed impotence and one retrograde ejaculation. Again, a certain number of changes in sexual function after surgery may not be specific to prostatic surgery. In general, those patients who tended to retain sexual activity were younger and more likely to be free of diabetes or of hypertension requiring therapy.

THE PHYSICIAN AND PATIENT TALK

It has not been unknown for professionals, physicians and even urologists to tell a patient flatly that he will be impotent after certain procedures. This can produce an iatrogenic impotence. It is not always the urologist who makes this mistake, it may be the referring physician, other professionals as well as a friend, gossip or the patient's own confusion.

It is tempting to quote the frequency charts of Kinsey or those developed in a similar manner where large numbers of patients seen in private practice were surveyed. These data provide a picture of declining frequency of sexual activity with age but the data are *not* useful in dealing with any one individual patient since individual psychological, physical and pathologic factors alter the picture greatly.[17]

Male erection and orgasm are largely a central nervous system and psychic phenomenon. Their preservation postoperatively is largely a function of the patient's previous sexual habits and intensity of interest. Hence, the consequences of transurethral, suprapubic and retropubic prostatectomy probably tend to fall more into the psychological rather than the urological realm.

A number of excellent research studies done seem to give support to this conclusion. Madorsky and co-workers[12] studied eighteen consecutive patients with a diagnosis of benign prostatic hypertrophy requiring transurethral prostatic resection. These patients averaged 65 years of age. Each patient underwent preoperative sleep studies. Of those who claimed to be sexually potent, two were impotent when penile plethysmography was performed. Of three who said they were impotent, one had nocturnal erections.

Four weeks following transurethral resection of the prostate, they were again studied with penile plethysmography. Seven had erections of shorter duration while seven showed increased duration of erections. There was no postoperative loss of complete penile erection and no significant differences could be detected in comparing pre- and postoperative potency. Three patients stated they had improved erections, four complained of decreased potency. No one complained of entire loss of erection.

Finkle and Moyers[4] reported that 50 per cent of 101 men were potent preoperatively, and irrespective of whether the perineal, transurethral, suprapubic or even retropubic operative route was used, 69 per cent of these remained potent; 66 per cent of 29 patients undergoing perineal prostatectomy retained potency. This bore out the conclusion of Lee et al.[10] following 3400 prostatectomies, that no one prostatic operation has a monopoly on being blamed for impotence!

In a subsequent study by Finkle and Moyers,[5] they reported that of 30

patients who had undergone open perineal biopsy and elective prostatectomy, only 7 became impotent postoperatively.

Gold and Hotchkiss[7] confirmed by questionnaire that the incidence of
diminished potency post-prostatectomy was related more to age than to
type of prostatectomy. These workers defined potency as ability to activate psychic desire for sexual intercourse sufficiently for penile erection and adequately for coitus, and to achieve gratification, usually
ejaculation, during the sexual act any time within the past year.

The older literature reflected a pervasive assumption in our society
that individuals over 50 should no longer be sexually active and that
prostatectomy was merely the final step. Those urologists who took
pains to preserve their patients' potency were viewed as humoring their
patients, and those patients who reported continuing potency were
viewed as unusual.

In 1959, Finkle and co-workers[3] studied 101 ambulatory male patients
between ages 55 and 86. Fifty patients had had coitus in the past year,
although twice as many of those below 70 were sexually active when
compared to those above 70. They found that the availability of a partner
was the most influential factor in determining frequency of intercourse.
This work was ahead of its time and received inadequate attention.

Errors have thus crept into the literature because attempts were made
to assess impotence, potency and sexual activity postoperatively without
having recorded a preoperative baseline.

OTHER CONDITIONS AFFECTING SEXUALITY

It must not be overlooked that specific sexual dysfunctions such as
premature ejaculation and severe psychological impotence may occur in
patients undergoing prostatectomy. These must be treated psychologically and will require specific sexual, marital or dual sex therapy. Surgical patients are not exempt from psychopathology unrelated to the
surgery.

Pre-prostatectomy vasectomy is occasionally performed to minimize
the possibility of retrograde infection of the epididymis. There has been
abundant experience with vasectomy for sterilization and it is well established that vasectomy does not interfere with potency. Impotence
following vasectomy is psychological until proven otherwise. Inter-
estingly, a historical survey has shown that vasectomy has been used
both to treat impotence and to attempt to produce it.[6]

Hematospermia is the appearance of blood in the ejaculate. Its incidence is increased in patients with benign prostatic hypertrophy. It is
an alarming symptom which rarely is due to any serious disease. It is
usually due to the rupture of a small blood vessel during ejaculation in

the seminal vesicle or along the ejaculatory path and requires reassurance and no therapy.

A few words must be added about the management of other medical and surgical conditions which may co-exist in patients undergoing prostatectomy. It is not always the prostatectomy and its symptoms that interfere with sexual function. Medical problems such as diabetes, heart disease, arthritis, among others, and emotional problems such as depression all are known to interfere to some extent with sexuality. The dosages of certain drugs used in the treatment of hypertension, epilepsy, depression and other conditions must be re-examined in the light of their effect upon potency. Alternative drugs, if available, should be recommended to the patient's physician.

Impotence occurs occasionally as a complication of urethral laceration or from fractured pelvis. Waterhouse and co-workers[18] have reported that resection of the symphysis pubis in order to facilitate the operative approach to the urethra for the treatment of stricture did not produce impotence in 16 patients. More likely, the impotence reported after severe pelvic fracture and associated urethral stricture may be due either to a non-specific effect of the serious trauma and the invalidism produced thereby, or to damage to the nerve supply in the pelvis essential for penile erection (in a manner analogous to the operative dissection).

Peyronie's disease, manifest by hard, thickened and even calcified plaques of degenerating tissue in the shaft of the penis, may or may not interfere with penile function. Many more patients have this disease than know it and it is often discovered accidently. A small number of patients have pain, penile curvature and sexual disability due to the deformity. Impotence, however, is a common complaint. There is no clear-cut correlation between the degree of disease, deformity or pain and the degree of impotence; some patients complain of the curvature interfering with actual intromission, while others complain of the impotence.

Peyronie's, although a chronic disease, is considered self-limiting. It has its own psychological aspects with respect to potency. It is not related to prostatectomy, except as a coincidental finding.

The concept of the male climacteric is vague and controversial. Malin[13] sees it as a definite but rare clinical entity. The climacteric male experiences the same symptom complex as does the menopausal female. There is a marked elevation of urinary male hormone secretion and testicular atrophy with resultant loss of libido and impotence. The male climacteric does respond to injections of male hormone. It is important to note, however, that the male climacteric is not considered a normal part of the aging process.

COUNSELING THE PROSTATECTOMY PATIENT

The patient being considered for prostatectomy should be questioned in order to establish his prior level of sexual activity. This should be compared with the level of sexual activity prior to the onset of his illness and to the needs, desires and demands of his partner if he has one.

A sexual as well as medical history is both a diagnostic and a therapeutic instrument. Unless the proper questions are asked, the professional does not obtain the necessary information. It is during the history that communication between doctor and patient commences and management really begins.

The doctor must detect those who have been sexually inactive early in life and those who are sexually inactive because of other disabilities. He must locate the fears, misconceptions and partner problems which the patient may be reluctant to reveal. He should encourage the patient to voice his fears and questions.

A good medical history will also reveal whether the patient is taking drugs for hypertension, depression or cardiac disease which may interfere with sexual functioning. Self-imposed restrictions and beliefs, religious orthodoxy or emotional inhibition can be detected. It has been found that when a proper history is taken, many of the misconceptions and fears can be handled immediately, promptly and simply. They may disappear in a sigh of relief or fade away leaving a very grateful, less harried or haggard patient.

Zohar and co-workers[20] selected 15 of 104 consecutive prostatectomy patients who were under 70 years of age, presently married, potent at a preoperative interview and who had histologic findings only of benign prostatic hyperplasia. Seven of the patients had a special explanation of the forthcoming operation, the anesthesia, ward routines and the postoperative course as well as the operation itself. They were reassured that preoperative sexual capacity would be maintained except for dry orgasm and that no other impairment of function would occur. The others received no explanation at all. Not one of the seven who were reassured suffered impotence; but 5 of the 8 who did not receive any explanation suffered postoperative impotence. Although a small pilot study, this is an exceedingly important one. It makes the point that **a careful history, time spent on preoperative explanation, as well as support and reassurance are very important to postoperative sexual function.**

Adequate counseling can prevent and reduce sexual disability. The counselor must dispel myths and ignorance, particularly those propagated by well-meaning friends and relatives. He must deal with the fears due to misinformation and false expectation and the fears created by the silence of professionals. He must anticipate the patient's unspoken questions.

150

It is important for the professional to assess the prior degrees of sexual activity of the patient. As already pointed out, many men who report impotence postoperatively have been impotent or inactive for years prior to surgery.

The availability of a partner must be considered. It is important to determine whether the patient is single, widowed or divorced. The professional must understand that single, widowed or divorced does not necessarily mean sexually inactive. One must learn the state of his wife's health, her sexual appetite, the presence or absence of any disabilities and her willingness, desire and interest in sexuality.

It is necessary to assess the patient's emotional reaction to his sexual life, whether he has excessive Victorianism, religious orthodoxy, inhibitions, fears, anxieties or a general level of dissatisfaction.

The professional must be alert to signs of misconceptions, confusions and myths regarding sexual function. The specific myth that prostatectomy is a serious, potentially fatal operation is a misconception harking back to the early part of the century. It can create unnecessary fear and anxiety and affect the operative result.

It is important to describe to the patient the various diagnostic procedures which he must undergo, such as rectal examination, cystoscopy, intravenous urograms, enemas, multiple physical examinations, the need to wear a catheter postoperatively for several days, the need to restore a normal urinary habit, the need for parenteral medications and other special treatments.

Just as in pediatric practice, adult patients need to be briefed as to what to expect, so that groundless or conjured fears do not complicate their convalescence or hospital course. The more intelligent, aggressive or inquisitive patients will demand this information. All patients deserve it.

It is important to enlist the patient's cooperation in the spirit of early ambulation, from instructing him to move and take deep breaths immediately upon awakening from anesthesia, to walking on the day of or after surgery to resume early ambulation and later on, to resume sexual activity.

In this manner, positive expectations are implanted early, objectively, realistically and rationally. Much preventive psychotherapy is accomplished with little effort when the patient is told concretely that *there will be a tomorrow,* that the prostatectomy only *temporarily* interrupts his sexual life.

The law now demands that patients receive "informed consent" information. This means that the patient must be presented with all the various alternatives of therapy and each major diagnostic intervention, and warned as to all the relevant consequences, sequelae and complications, as well as the benefits and indications. Patients often turn to the doctor and say, "Please, you decide." In one way or another, they look to the physician to make the decision. Urologists must gently lead the patient to make the decision, even as he indicates clearly to the patient which way he thinks the decision should go. The doctor finds himself to be adviser, counselor and friend but he cannot legally be the only decision maker. Should there be a poor result, an unhappy or dissatisfied or disgruntled patient, or a dispute postoperatively, the burden will fall on the operating urologist to show that the decision and choice were the patient's.

In the frame of reference depicted, the expectations of the patient, the urologist, the spouse, the family and the nurse, the office or hospital staff must be realistic and optimistic. Depending on the personality, cultural level, and degree of realism of the patient, one must present the positive expectations in a comprehensible manner. The patient must be given the message that he will recover in spite of the temporary dysfunction and disability and that his sexual function will return soon after his urinary function.

THERAPY FOR POST-PROSTATECTOMY IMPOTENCE

Much can be done for some prostatectomy patients who are impotent. They may need instruction in normal changes in sexual function consonant with aging. This may require subsequent changes in the mechanics of sexuality, the extension of foreplay, adequate sensual and manual stimulation by each partner, acceptance of varied positions for intercourse, the proper use of lubricants and gynecological consultation for his sexual partner.

For the patient who becomes totally impotent and who does not respond to psychological treatment, two types of penile prostheses are currently available: the Small-Carrion silastic prosthesis and the Scott inflatable prosthesis. These prostheses have been implanted with a satisfactorily low complication rate.

The Scott inflatable implantable prosthesis requires compression of a small implanted scrotal bulb to produce the erection. It is more nearly physiologic than the Small-Carrion prosthesis, which remains rigid permanently. The former does carry a higher re-operation rate than does the Small-Carrion. Research in this area is active. Experience and acceptance are growing.

Adequate sexual function in the prostatectomy patient must be defined in terms of the larger perspectives of sex: in the pleasure of companionship, by sensuality and eroticism, by touch and foreplay, by mutuality of partner satisfaction, as well as by the usual trio of erection, ejaculation and orgasm. Sexual function does not stop for many patients because fertility ceases.

This broad concept of sexual function actually benefits the patient. Satisfactions lost in one area due to disease or aging can be compensated by satisfactions retained or regained in other aspects of broadly defined sexuality. The most important principle to remember is that neither prostatectomy nor aging per se need result in impotence.

REFERENCES

1. Caine, M., Pfau, A. and Perlberg, S. The use of alpha-adrenergics in benign prostatic obstruction. Brit. J. Urol. 48:255, 1976.
2. Ellis, W.J. and Grayhack, J.T. Sexual function in aging males after orchiectomy and estrogen therapy. J. Urol. 89:895, 1963.
3. Finkle, A.L., Moyers, T.G. et al. Sexual potency in aging males. I. Frequency of coitus among clinical patients. JAMA 170:1391, 1959.
4. Finkle, A.L. and Moyers, T.B. Sexual potency in aging males. IV. Status of prostatectomy patients before and after prostatectomy. J. Urol. 84:152, 1960.
5. Finkle, A.L. and Moyers, T.B. Sexual potency in aging males. V. Coital ability following open perineal prostatic biopsy. J. Urol. 84:649, 1960.
6. Gee, W.F. A history of surgical treatment of impotence. Urol. 3: 1975.
7. Gold, F.M. and Hotchkiss, R.S. Sexual potency following simple prostatectomy. N.Y. State J. Med. 2987, 1969.
8. Herr, H.W. Preservation of Sexual Potency in Prostatic Cancer Patients after Pelvic Lymphadenectomy and Iodine 125 Implant. Amer. Urol. Assoc. Convention, May 1978, Washington, D.C.
9. Kinsey, A.C., Pomeroy, W.B. and Martin, C.E. Sexual Behavior in the Human Male. Philadelphia, W.B. Saunders, 1948.
10. Lee, W.L., Malashock, E.M. and Davis, N.B. Experience with transurethral prostatic resection and perineal prostatectomy in one clinic: A comparative review of 3400 patients. Tr. Soc. So. Cent. Sect. AUA: 56, 1957.
11. Lytton, B., Emery, J.M. and Harvard, B.M. The incidence of benign prostatic obstruction. J. Urol. 99:639, 1968.
12. Madorsky, M.L., Ashamalla, M.G. et al. Post-prostatectomy impotence. J. Urol. 115:401, 1976.
13. Malin, J.M. Sex after urologic surgery and informed consent. Med. Trial Tech. Quart. 21:35, 1974.
14. Masters, W. and Johnson, V. Human Sexual Response. Boston, Little Brown, 1965.
15. Melchior, J., Valk, W. et al. Transurethral prostatectomy. J. Urol. 112:634, 1974.
16. O'Conor, V.J., Jr. Suprapubic Prostatectomy. In Urology, Vol. 3 (Campbell and Harrison, Eds.) Philadelphia, W.B. Saunders, 1970, p. 2405.
17. Pearlman, C.K. and Kobashi, L.I. Frequency of intercourse in men. J. Urol.: 298, 1972.
18. Waterhouse, K., Abrams, J.I. and Negro, P. Wedge resection of symphysis pubis for stricture. J. Urol. 111:188, 1974.
19. Windle, R. and Roberts, J.B.M. Ejaculatory function after prostatectomy. Proc. Roy. Soc. Med. 67:1160, 1974.
20. Zohar, J., Meiraz, D. et al. Factors influencing sexual activity after prostatectomy. J. Urol. 116:332, 1976.

13

Sexual Consequences of Gynecological Operations

DENNIS J. MASSLER, M.D., MONA M. DEVANESAN, M.D., FACOG

INTRODUCTION

Gynecological procedures ought not be dismissed with cursory explanations and a physician's half-hearted attempts to elicit patients' fears and feelings. The preoperative appointments are important to the success of the service. The necessity of exposing the patient's fantasy of what will be done to her body and the sequelae regarding her capacity to function as a woman is beyond question. Accurate information, coupled with the dispelling of myths, as well as the opportunity to interact with an approachable empathetic surgeon can minimize the potential emotional traumata. The exchange between doctor and patient at this early preoperative stage can help the patient mobilize and erect efficient and effective defenses and satisfactory compensatory behaviors. She can then incorporate this necessary operation or procedure into the context of her life without radically upsetting her psychic equilibrium.

The physician's implicit belief that his patient is and will continue to be a sexual being, coupled with explicit advice regarding postoperative sexual response promotes a positive sexual result.

Whatever the gynecologic procedure contemplated or scheduled, the sooner the husband or significant other can be incorporated into the discussion, the better—while the patient herself needs time to assess what the experience will mean to her physically and psychologically, in order to go through any necessary emotional adjustments and defensive maneuvers. Partner participation will help lessen the likelihood of con-

154

scious or unconscious antagonism of her spouse and decrease the potential of her feeling left alone to deal with this crucial life experience.

A woman's sense of self is biologically based, societally and parentally nurtured, culturally and relationally reinforced. That there is a biologic, genetic, endocrine difference between male and female children is clear by birth. From birth onward, from the moment the genitals are seen, and male infants are deposited into blue and female into pink, parents and society collaborate to expand and nurture the inherent differences and to introduce new learned differences. Cultural attitudes and beliefs coupled with the interaction between the maturing girl and her peers (and later her boyfriends) reinforce her concepts of self and of womanhood. In most cases, the final product is a person whose sense of self-esteem is based on motherhood, femininity, and the capacity to attract and maintain a relationship with a man.

The awareness of a difference between boys' and girls' genitals occurs early with many behaviors, privileges, sanctions, and feelings attributed to these differences. A girl's genitals begin to take on special meanings which are modified and/or reinforced through the time of puberty, when menses occurs and the first dramatic evidence that her uterus exists is manifested. The symbolic meanings of her buttocks, vagina, breasts, skin, uterus, clitoris, etc. exist on many levels. Some of the importance attached to these organs is related to their actual functions; some is related to the beliefs, biases, and emotional transpositions which occur during the maturation process.

The womb holds specific emotional import to a female. It figures in a wealth of positive experiences in which she has been or will be involved. In an attempt to identify herself with her mother and accept herself as a woman, her childhood was spent playing with dolls, playing house, and learning to correlate being a mother with being a woman. The womb later becomes associated with converting the childhood play into the adult reality of motherhood as an essential element of femaleness.

Menstruation, although associated with capacity to bear children, and evidence that there is a uterus, takes on other psychically important functions. It is proof positive that a change has occurred and that the girl has begun her journey into womanhood. For some women, the cyclic nature of menses has far-reaching associations in her life, and its occurrence or cessation is often linked to vigor, energy, and cleanliness among other things. Some women view the uterus as a sexual organ and believe that it is essential to sexual response. In this context, it is tied closely to her feelings of attractiveness and sexual desirability.

The ovaries, also internal though more directly associated with specific sexual functioning, are viewed in a similar light. In reality, the ovaries play a valuable role in the production of hormones essential for sexual response. They help keep the vagina supple and soft as well as facilitate lubrication via their estrogenic effect.

The ovaries are also often associated with the womb, and play an important role in the woman's sense of self, especially as related to specific motherhood, womanhood, and femininity. These are, however, less often perceived as sexual organs.

The vagina is not essential to sexual response, as there are many ways of relating sexually without a functioning vagina. Despite this, from a physical point of view, any operation or procedure which would compromise the utility of the vagina could have a severe impact on a woman's capacity to have and enjoy sex. The vagina is seen by males and females alike as the specific sexual contact organ in the woman. A great many people believe that making love is only worthwhile when the penetration, the enveloping of the penis—an engulfing and penetration of one's partner—is achieved.

Though the clitoris is the trigger for orgasm in the female, the attractiveness and utility of the vagina is often perceived as more important. It is seen as the organ used to invite, accept and entertain a man's sexual advances. Its odor or fragrance is important in a woman's sexual self-perception. Any procedure resulting in narrowing, shortening, hardening, or in any other way impairing the function or appearance of the vagina could result in dyspareunia and could effect sexual desire.

It was not until the work of Masters and Johnson that the clitoris got the recognition it deserved. Subsequent to their dispelling the mythical difference between clitoral and vaginal orgasm, there has been a growing awareness and interest on the part of many women in the function and pleasure associated with this organ. It is not essential to sexual interaction, but it serves as an important facilitator of female sexual response and pleasure, (though not tied to reproduction) motherhood, femininity, or desirability. It would also play a great role in minimizing sexual desire or pleasure if anything were to impair its functioning and orgasmic dysfunction were to ensue.

The vulva is often depicted artistically as a flower. It is perceived as the female genital organ, and its attractiveness is of considerable importance to a woman and her partner. Besides the psychic importance of the labia and introitus, there is an important physical concern. Since this is generally the gate to specific sexual interaction, anything which results in pain, displeasure, embarrassment or concern centering around the introitus can have far-reaching effects. Pain can result in dyspareunia and vaginismus; embarrassment, shame, or anxiety can have a similar effect, as well as decrease libido.

GENERAL COUNSELING CONCEPTS

The least a patient should expect of her doctor is that each of us be aware of our own attitudes and limitations. A comfortable and flexible physician is the most capable of eliciting the fears, misconceptions and concerns of his patient. We can take our patients' questions seriously even if they are not fully understandable to us when first verbalized. We can provide enough time to allow verbalization of questions and concerns. This might not be realistic during busy office hours, but time set aside before or after hours could be extremely advantageous for the patient and might better enable us to incorporate their partners into our counseling.

It is important to provide an approachable, willing and listening ear. Special attention needs to be paid to a patient's fantasies of what is going on in her body, what the procedure will be like and most important, what the results of the procedure will be. Her preoperative fantasy of how the procedure will affect her emotionally, physically and sexually can greatly influence her recovery. If the questions regarding the sexual, relationship, reproductive, physiologic, and emotional outcome of the operation are elicited preoperatively, the physician will have the time and opportunity to provide advice and education which can serve to lessen or mitigate any misconceptions and misunderstandings. Honest reassurance of normalcy and capability of full or limited sexual functioning will go a long way if begun preoperatively, it incorporates the partner, and is tailored to the individual couple's situation and concerns. Attention paid to helping the patient and her partner communicate openly about sexual feelings, concerns, desires and fears is often helpful and frequently easier in the hands of a trusted physician postoperatively if the doors of communication are opened preoperatively. Since time is required to adjust to the inevitable changes, preparing the patient well in advance of the particular procedure is likely to yield cooperation and fewer sexual and relationship problems. Merely allowing the couple to verbalize sexual feelings, concerns and questions openly is a liberating experience for many couples, especially if joined with permission and suggestions of ways to experiment sexually.

Privacy and confidentiality are obviously imperative. Allocation of specific time for a specific couple without the usual distractions of a busy practice is vital.

Clarity in explanations and advice is essential. It is also important that the source of the information is made clear: whether it is medically accepted fact, a result of personal observation, or a suggestive assumption. An explanation of the need for the procedure finally executed leads to less psychological and sexual sequelae. It eliminates misunder-

standing and the possible erosion of trust, resulting in the physician in-
advertently disqualifying himself as a supporting agent during the
process of illness, surgery and recovery. Involving the patient in the
decision-making process regarding her own health helps prepare her to
accept the results. (The physician is at his best when viewing himself as
an adviser rather than a decision-maker.) The responsibility of the gynecologist is to use proper medical judgment, obtain informed consent
and to unearth present or potential problems in many areas, including
sexual functioning. It is his/her responsibility to treat, consult or refer
appropriately depending upon his skills and inclinations, as well as the
constraints of time. Though it is usually preferable for the gynecologist
to do his/her own counseling, since a trusting therapeutic alliance has
already been established, there are times when the emotional discomfort, psychopathology, or relationship difficulties are such that the expertise, time, or inclination of the gynecologist would best be served by
an appropriate request for consultative assistance or referral. Regardless of the physician's predisposition toward or against treating and/or
counseling the patient sexually, it is necessary to focus on the sexual
aspect of the patient's life relating to the upcoming procedure in the
same way he would be concerned with a patient's capacity to return to
her usual household activities.

HYSTERECTOMY

Misconceptions

The terms *subtotal* and *total hysterectomy* may mean different things
to the patient than to the physician. A subtotal hysterectomy is defined
as the removal of the body of the uterus with retention of the cervix,
fallopian tubes and ovaries. Total hysterectomy is defined as the removal of the uterus and cervix. Total hysterectomy with the removal of
tubes and ovaries is called total abdominal hysterectomy with bilateral
salpingo-oophorectomy. To the layman, total hysterectomy may mean
anything up to and including removal of uterus, vagina, ovaries, tubes;
thus a total "cleaning out." Partial hysterectomy may be construed as the
removal of just the uterus and cervix, or a piece of the uterus—or it may
evoke some other erroneous picture or fantasy.

Some patients take for granted that menstruation will continue after
a hysterectomy. It can be a shock when they find they cannot and will
not menstruate. To some women, menstruation is a period of their cyclic lives when the poisons which have built up in their systems are
eliminated. Douglas observed the belief among Puerto Rican patients at
Bellevue Hospital that symptoms of pre-menstrual tension represent the
accumulation of some poison in the system. "They believe that when

they no longer menstruate the material is backed up and they will be uncomfortable in the indefinite future."[26] The cleansing function of the menstrual flow may be perceived as being brought to an end with the performance of a hysterectomy and there may be resultant fears that the poisons will accumulate.

Menses is seen by some women as a time of renewing vigor and energy. The cycle may be seen in terms of build-up and release of tension, as giving a rhythm to life, and as an organized pattern that regulates daily activities. For these women, hysterectomy may signal the end of their normal cyclicity, and with its loss the end of a source of energy, strength, youth and well-being, as well as the loss of the regulator of general body health.[27]

The picture in some women's minds when confronted with the concept of hysterectomy is that a void, a hole, or unfilled space or cavity is left where the womb used to be. Their misconceptions regarding anatomic sizes and organ proximities may contribute to irrational fears. In conjunction with this set of myths is the possibility that the hysterectomy patient may fear that her partner will be able to tell during intercourse that she has no uterus or that sex will feel different to her or to him. Some women fear that hysterectomy will cause sex to be diminished or abolished. This is borne out in the literature by the many reports of post-hysterectomy sexual abstinence.

Another myth is that the removal of this bad or unwanted organ which has caused so many symptoms and so much discomfort will not only result in a cure of the specific symptoms, but will also result in a successful cure of pre-existing sexual or relationship dysfunctions. Some women have unreasonably grandiose expectations regarding the potential benefit of their hysterectomy.

Anatomical, Psychiatric and Functional Sequelae

In reality, the organic sequelae of hysterectomy are quite limited, though worthy of the physician's consideration. Current medical knowledge suggests that no major influence on libido, excitement, lubrication and orgasm is exerted physiologically as a result of total or partial hysterectomy. This information needs to be emphasized to the patient.

Some of the literature does suggest a possible endocrine imbalance following hysterectomy which evokes the question of whether future research will demonstrate an endocrine function in connection with the uterus.[80] Field and Field concluded that, even in the presence of both ovaries, there are vasomotor changes secondary to hysterectomy which may be related to possible endocrine function of the uterus.[33]

When a wide cuff is removed, as for carcinoma in situ or carcinoma of the cervix, the result can be a shorter vagina or a narrower vaginal barrel. Masters and Johnson state, "Physicians, when performing hysterectomy, may overlook the fact that the cervix enters the vagina through the superior wall of that organ."[61] Deep thrusting by the partner against the scar tissue may lead to pain on intercourse, months or even years after surgery. Because of the time lag, the operating surgeon may never be aware of the acquired dyspareunia. The patient might best be served by her surgeon if an attempt is made to keep the resultant scar away from the axis of deep thrusting.

Close to one million hysterectomies are performed every year in the United States, for reasons which range from cancer to contraception. The question as to whether hysterectomy should be limited to cancerous organs has been approached from many sides. At one extreme, Wright states, "The uterus has one function—after the last planned pregnancy, the uterus becomes a useless, bleeding, symptom-producing, potentially cancer-bearing organ, and therefore should be removed."[101] This point of view sees elective hysterectomy as prophylactic, providing symptomatic relief. He feels that it will enable women to live more comfortable lives, free of not only the potentially dangerous or lethal problems which can occur in the genital tract, but also the monthly problems, and the anxieties of possible pregnancy. Short of that position there are many authors who feel that emotional disorders, marital problems and sexual compaints are unrelated to hysterectomy. For instance, in large studies, Ackner and Melody concur that women with postoperative emotional disturbances had emotional disturbances preoperatively.[2,63]

Even on this side of the spectrum dissent can be found, however. Donahue states, "An operation that results in complications for 30 to 45 of every 100 women receiving it, and is followed by death of 1 woman in 500 to 1000 can be considered to have considerable somatic impact that can have major psychological reactions."[25] According to Gallo, "Hysterectomy injures the patient psychologically only in proportion to her ignorance." If she clearly understands that she only loses her reproductive capacity but remains absolutely normal in other respects, the injury is minimal.[36] In a study by Drellich et al.,[28] the other side of the issue is represented admirably by the quotation: "Hysterectomy is a matter of great consequence in the life of a woman. It is apparent that the uniquely female organs are greatly valued and are seen as very important in maintaining the total adaptation of the woman." They state that the uterus is valued as a childbearing, cleansing instrument, as a sexual organ, source of strength, youth and feminine attractiveness, as well as a regulator of general body health and well-being. They also suggest that anxieties surrounding the imminent loss of this valued organ are responsible for delays in treatment and irrational preoperative fears and can contribute to prolonged postoperative invalidism.[27]

By the World Health Organization standards, health is not just a state of absence of disease, but one of physical, emotional and social well-being. Part of the social role of the female concerns her biologic capability of reproduction, and thus sexual intercourse. Her capacity to carry out the role is dependent on the health of her reproductive organs, as well as on her sense of self-identity. This identity is correlated with her attractiveness and sexual desirability to a great extent, and her ability to bear children. This makes her breasts, vagina, uterus, clitoris, ovaries, etc. essential to her adaptation and self-assessment as a woman, as well as her sense of appreciation and acceptance by others.

There is an emotional response to any physical assault on the body. The magnitude of the response is expected to be proportional to the degree of emotional investment one has in the part of the body being assaulted. Ruth Benedict states, "Sharp, sudden, and irreversible cultural or physical changes necessitating some alteration in a person's social roles and expectations may result in a breakdown in normal functioning. The more sudden the impact, the less preparation for it, the more disturbing the effect."[11] Sanford Wolf goes so far as to say, "Hysterectomy is equal to surgical disruption of the self-concept of femininity."[99] Hysterectomy is an obviously irreversible surgical procedure and by its very nature and social definition, is connected with three important female functions: motherhood, womanhood, and femininity. Melody states, "The social roles available to an individual, as well as one's body image, self-concept or self-evaluation, are to a large degree determined by the social contact organs and their symbolic meaning to the individual."[63]

Barglow and his associates did a study entitled "Pseudocyesis and Psychiatric Sequelae of Sterilization," pairing up women who had undergone hysterectomy and tubal ligation.[6] They divided their group into three co-sterilization groups. Group I was psychologically healthy, had few somatic symptoms, and patient fantasies and defenses correlated with working through object loss. They exhibited a gradual shift of emotional energy from the reproductive task to other life activities, much like successful mourning work resulting in a new ego-body integration without childbearing function. Patients with diagnosis of cancer of the cervix, uterus, or ovaries may experience least difficulty in mourning the loss of the organs since these are now viewed as bad, undesirable or life-threatening organs. Group II were immature, impulse-ridden and hysterical. As Theresa Benedek recognized, pregnancy may be an immense source of narcissistic supplies and the fetus itself may be a substitute for the gratification of outside object relationships.[10] In this group the pregnant woman in her placid, vegetative calmness enjoys her pregnant body, which is like a reservoir replenished with libidinal feelings.[12] They fear loss of love or super-ego sanctions causing guilt, shame and conversion symptoms including pseudocyesis. Group III women spent most of their energy in denial of the sterilization. The result was incapacitating pelvic illness immediately following sterilization. They perceived themselves as damaged and mutilated by the operation which resulted in a regression to the state of primitive oral fears. Physical illness or separation were important contributing factors. Loss of an important sexual function was perceived as a threat of damage to the body integrity, and the response of the patient was to deny the absence of childbearing capacity. Loss of an organ whose presence is reaffirmed monthly cannot easily be denied. Painful pelvic symptoms represented the presence of body parts or functions which were necessary for repair of damaged body integrity. (Their unconscious self-explanation is that since the pain hurts, the part is therefore present.) Barglow concluded that tubal ligation had better long-term psychological consequences than did hysterectomy.[6]

Some women look at sterilization as the permanent relief of fears of getting pregnant during coitus which results in more relaxed and spontaneous loving. Neil et al. reported an improvement in the sex life of 50 per cent of sterilized women compared with 74 per cent of women whose husbands had been sterilized. Both of these figures are correlated with a secure form of contraception.[73] The results can go either way, with some women reporting an increase in sexual problems, i.e., decrease in libido secondary to loss of childbearing ability, while others have a decrease in sexual problems and an increase in sexual libido.

Douglas states, "Menstruation is sometimes seen as giving rhythm to life in an organized pattern that would set regulated daily activities."[26] It is the first visible sign of the presence of a woman's uterus corroborating its existence. It is seen as an excretory organ, a regulator of sexual functioning, work schedule, and social life. Some women are generally glad to be rid of messy bleeding, mood swings and activity cycling that accompanies the menstrual cycle. For some, menstruation is desirable because they attribute their sickly behavior to it. Yet some see menses as the "curse" or "plague" or the "mess" and view menses as monthly cleansing causing an increase in vigor, energy, and healthy normalcy.

Repeated and controlled studies indicate that hysterectomy can cause rejection by male partners, hot flushes (even with conservation of ovarian tissue), severe hot flushes (following ovariectomy), weight changes, painful intercourse, lingering fatigue, prolonged convalescence, depression, sleep disturbances, and long-term psychourinary problems.

Psychourinary Problems

Richards' study indicated a high rate of urinary problems in hysterectomized women compared with his control group. Utilizing a 30-month follow-up, he found a high incidence of stress incontinence as well as nocturnal frequency at a statistically significant level of .001.[80] In Dodd's study of weight changes of 108 women past the age of 40 without ovaries, 54 per cent had gained under ten pounds, 18 per cent under twenty pounds, and 18 per cent under thirty pounds.[24] Ackner's study showed that 38 per cent gained weight while 14 per cent lost weight.[2] Dalton found that 50 per cent had an increase of 14 pounds in one year and 35 per cent had gained at least 28 pounds in one year; he concluded that acute weight gain occurs during the first two or three months followed by a gradual, persistent rise.[18]

Hot Flushes

Hot flushes were found to be common when ovaries were left in the abdominal cavity. According to Richards, "The most probable variable factor which suggests itself is interference with the ovarian blood supply at operation."[80] In studies on humans and other mammals undergoing hysterectomy, there was strong indication that removal of the uterus has a measurable effect on gonadal activity. This was supported by Stone and co-workers[89] as well as by Andreoli.[4]

Fatigue

In Drellich and Bieber's study,[27] over half of the patients studied experienced weakness, loss of strength and easy fatigability which was corroborated by Richards' study in which 54 per cent of the hysterectomized and 13 per cent of the controls also had excessive tiredness.[81]

The most widely studied emotional effect of hysterectomy was depression. Steiner and Aleksandrowicz compared the effects of hysterectomy and cholecystectomy and found the incidence of depression to be three times greater for hysterectomy.[87] Bragg studied 1601 patients with hysterectomy versus 1162 cholecystectomy patients and found the hysterectomy patients to be at a three times greater risk for first psychiatric admission to a hospital. Once admitted, they remained hospitalized five times longer than those who had undergone cholecystectomy.[12] Barker also studied hysterectomy versus gallbladder surgery; he found a 2½-time higher incidence of psychiatric referral for hysterectomy versus cholecystectomy patients (whose referral rate is itself three times as great as the general population). He found the peak period for psychiatric referral was in the second year post-hysterectomy, 85 per cent of which was for depression.[9] Referrals for women with normal uteri were twice as high as for those with an abnormal uterus. Divorced and separated women as well as those with previous psychiatric histories were at higher risk. Richards found 33 per cent of hysterectomized patients versus 7 per cent of the controls to be depressed, with the mean duration of the depression 24.6 months versus 10.9 for controls.[81] Raphael found 60 per cent of her sample to have post-hysterectomy "blues" as opposed to 20 per cent of the gallbladder patients.[78] Melody lists three types of candidates for post-operative depression: 1) the polysurgery addict or hysterical neurotic; 2) the post-hysterectomy depressive (whom he referred to as "the indifferent woman"); and 3) the over-anxious woman who worries about everything.[63] Both Barker[9] and Richards[80] believe that hysterectomy is associated with a greater need for medications to treat anxiety or depression, or to seek psychiatric help, and is most likely to be manifested during the second year post-surgically. Hampton and Tarnasky[39] add that there seems to be less emotional disturbance associated with tubal ligation. Normally the period for mourning loss of a valued object is 6 to 8 weeks following the loss and the grief period is usually completed within 6 months.

If the husband or partner is distant, detached, or if he sees the patient as less sexually attractive, she is more likely to become depressed than if he is emotionally supportive and understanding and continues to find intercourse enjoyable or improved. This is supported by the studies of Melody,[63] Roeske,[84] Dennerstein et al.[20] and D'Escopo.[22] Some studies indicate that depression may occur even in the presence of partner support. Some men are dependent for their own identity on a woman's womb and need to support their own masculinity by maintaining the reproduction potential of the spouse—and hence their own.

The most frequent long-term psychopathologic reaction to hysterectomy is severe depression. Depression represents serious disruption of the female's role and identity. It reflects a woman's inability to reintegrate herself through the mourning process and re-establish significant relationships. Moore and Tulley concluded, as a result of their findings, that the term "post-hysterectomy depression" might be misleading, because it appears that the majority of first depressions developed prior to the operation.[70]

Effects on Sexual Functioning

In a report on 56 women who had undergone hysterectomy within five years of his study, Richards[80] found no consistent effect on or correlation with libido despite his finding that 70 per cent of the hysterectomized women had some increase in depression. However, 32 per cent of his subjects experienced a decrease in libido which he defines as less satisfaction or less frequent climax up to complete loss of desire; 45 per cent revealed no change, and 3 per cent had an increase in libido. Patterson and colleagues[76] found a 20 per cent increase in erotic drive, 60 per cent had no change, and 18 per cent reported a decrease. Horak[44] studied 139 patients with abdominal hysterectomy and 121 patients with vaginal hysterectomy and found no difference in sexuality between the two groups, nor any difference in rate of orgasm or libido before or after surgery. In his study, 180 of the 260 women had had orgasms preoperatively: 15 per cent reported an improvement in orgasms, 63 per cent noted no change, and 22 per cent reported a decline, but all continued to be orgasmic. He did, however, find that 20 of the women had no intercourse after the operation. Dalton[18] also found a higher rate of abstinence after hysterectomy, a whopping 42 per cent! Total hysterectomy performed vaginally or abdominally may cause a shortening of the vagina and leave scar tissue where the cervix is excised.

In the studies where patients were asked specifically whether sexual relations had changed following hysterectomy, the incidence of diminished sexual functioning varied from 10 per cent in Huffman's study[45] to 38 per cent in Richards' study.[81] Utian[94] found no correlation between sexual outcome and the conservation or destruction of ovarian function. Dennerstein et al.[20] reported a 37 per cent deterioration in sexual relations following hysterectomy, 34 per cent improvement, and 26 per cent unchanged, with no correlation found between administration of hormones and sexual dysfunction. "Sexual functioning" was defined as desire for sex, enjoyment of sex, ability to reach orgasm and ease of vaginal lubrication. They found that the single greatest preoperative concern was alteration in sexual functioning as a result of the operation. They also found that the worst sexual outcomes were seen in women who preoperatively had sexual frequency of less than once a week as opposed to those having had sexual intercourse more than once a week. The expectation that the operation would adversely affect sexual relations was correlated with deterioration in sexual relations postoperatively. These authors suggested that estrogen administration could be useful in preventing dyspareunia but probably would have no primary effect on sexual desire or enjoyment.

According to Richards,[81] sexuality has a biological and psychological base as indicated by the accentuation at puberty. Many women whose ovaries have been removed can and do enjoy coitus and report orgasms, but there are conflicting reports about the effect of the surgery on the strength of libido. In Richards' report, 35 per cent had decreased libido correlated with ovarian conservation and hysterectomy; 42 per cent had decreased libido with unilateral oophorectomy and hysterectomy; and 60 per cent had a decreased libido with bilateral oophorectomy and hysterectomy. Estrogen replacement does not replace androgens which are produced in ovaries. The role of the ovary in hormone production will be discussed later.

Sexual Counseling

Traditionally, women have been instructed to abstain from intercourse for six or more weeks following hysterectomy. There are no objective data to support this period of necessary abstinence, but most women do not demonstrate great emotional stress from this proscription if it is spelled out clearly. No data are available concerning the partner's response to this proscription.

It must be stated clearly that the proscription is *against introducing any foreign body into the vagina such as the penis, or applying pressure on the abdomen or placing stress on a fresh abdominal scar.* If the advice is "no sex"—this is often interpreted as advocating no sexual intimacy at all. The distinction needs to be made that hugging, kissing, petting, and mutual masturbation or desirable genital caressing is appropriate medically and desirable emotionally. A clear explanation of the reasons for the various instructions given is helpful. Pressure and strain on the healing abdominal wall may cause pain or adversely affect the healing process and hence must specifically be avoided.

Once the patient can tolerate a pelvic examination and has completely healed, which usually occurs by the fourth postoperative week, and the abdominal discomfort is minimal, the couple should be encouraged to re-establish fuller sexual activity. This must be evaluated at the postoperative examination. While early return to sexual intercourse can be encouraged, specific advice regarding coital positions is important. Initially, patients should be cautioned against deep and vigorous thrusting. Rear entry, or male superior with the woman's legs up against her chest wall should be avoided, as should any positions which would predispose toward deep thrusting. Suggested positions are the side-to-side, male superior with his legs outside his partner's, or female superior position.

Whenever the specific sexual activity, whether it be intercourse or not, becomes painful, it should be discontinued so as to prevent the establishment of a pattern of avoidance precipitated by the pain-producing stimulus. The object is to protect the patient from infection or any delay of the healing process and to minimize pain, while encouraging sexual activity. Most important, intimacy is never to be interrupted. It is extremely important in hysterectomy, as well as in any gynecologic procedure, to keep in mind the concept that *this is a sexually functional human being who often needs advice and attention concerning this vital realm of her life.* This aspect of the physician's responsibility preoperatively, operatively and postoperatively needs to be considered as a matter of course.

OOPHORECTOMY

Oophorectomy is the removal of the ovary, an organ which produces estrogens, progesterone, androgens and ova.

A bilateral oophorectomy is performed most often along with hysterectomy for ovarian or uterine malignancy, endometriosis and pelvic inflammatory disease. Occasionally the woman over forty is subjected to prophylactic removal of the ovaries. Proponents for prophylactic removal argue that within a decade the ovaries will undergo atrophy but always have the potential for malignant change.[38,86] Opponents present several arguments, including the low incidence of malignant change in ovaries retained after hysterectomy (0 to 2%);[79,97] and that the prophylactic removal of organs such as the testicles with their potential for malignant change is not accepted practice. Furthermore, the functions of the aging ovary may not be fully understood at present. Indeed, the postmenopausal ovaries are responsible for 50 per cent of the circulating plasma testosterone,[95] and their extirpation results in a small but significant decrease in circulating androstenedione.[48]

Misconceptions

One of the authors was referred a youthful-looking 30-year-old woman for loss of sexual desire. She had had a radical mastectomy and bilateral oophorectomy for cancer of the breast. She was in an emotionally supportive relationship. After a few sessions it became clear that the precipitating factor was not fear of death or the mutilating mastectomy procedure but an anxiety that she was rapidly going to shrivel up into an old woman subsequent to the oophorectomy. This is a concern of many women. Some women, as a method of denial, will misunderstand the procedure or forget the information given them.

Anatomical, Functional and Psychiatric Sequelae

Removal of ovarian tissue leaves the woman with a continuing supply of estrogen from adrenal sources. As a result of this, vaginal dryness and resultant dyspareunia is not a natural consequence until advancing years.

In a study of 100 patients followed after hysterectomy and bilateral

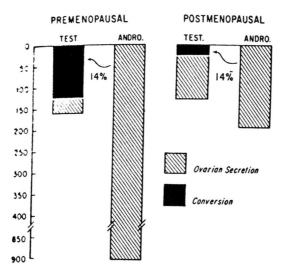

FIG. 1. Net fall of serum androstenedione and testosterone levels following oophorectomy in premenopausal and postmenopausal women. Striped portion represents ovarian secretion while solid portion depicts contribution from peripheral conversion of androstenedione. (From H.J. Judd, Clin. Obstet. Gynec., Vol. 19, Dec. 1976, p. 777.)

salpingo-oophorectomy for from 1 to 31 years, Chakravarti et al.[15] reported a fall in estradiol levels by 78 per cent below the mean values for day 1 to 10 of the menstrual cycle. The testosterone level fell by 27 per cent but stayed within the normal levels for the menstrual cycle. Judd graphically describes the testosterone and androstenedione changes following oophorectomy (Fig. 1).[49] The level of FSH (Follicular Stimulating Hormone) rose to a peak of 14 times the preoperative level after surgery and continued to be elevated for a longer period of time than after natural menopause. While 94 per cent of the oophorectomized women experienced vasomotor symptoms at one time or another, the symptoms subsided within five years in 92 per cent. In contrast, 74 per cent of 60 menopausal women experienced vasomotor symptoms.

Utian has concluded that hysterectomy has a deleterious effect on libido unrelated to estrogenic status and that psychological response cannot be excluded.[94] In Chakravarti's study[15] on endocrine changes and symptomatology following oophorectomy in premenopausal women, it was found that hysterectomy with bilateral oophorectomy resulted in depression in 62 per cent, insomnia in 48 per cent, loss of libido in 46 per cent, and dyspareunia in 38 per cent. Increasing apareunia was found with increasing age, and there were no significant differences correlated with the complaining subjects and blood levels of estradiol, testosterone, LH, or FSH. Thus, essentially, there were no psychogenic symptoms correlated with the level of any of the circulating hormones.[15]

Effects on Sexual Functioning

In lower animals there is often an identifiable positive relationship between sex hormones and sexual activity.

Judd and co-workers[48] found that ovariectomy in Rhesus monkeys abolished cyclic sexual activity and that hormone replacement restored the cycles. Ford and Beach,[34] in studies on lower mammals who were castrated, reported permanent elimination of sexual behavior in the females. On the other hand, adult chimpanzees with ovariectomy manifested a decrease in the frequency of coitus. They concluded that chimpanzees may permit sex to avoid injury. Ford and Beach stated, "Subhuman primates are not completely dependent on sex hormones to mate."

In a study of orgasmic frequency and plasma testosterone levels in normal human males, the mean testosterone levels were found to be higher for sexually less active men.[104] In a large study done on men by Monti et al.[69] there was an impressive lack of correlation between testosterone levels and questionnaire items related to sexual activity and interest. These researchers did, however, find a positive relationship between testosterone and current frequency of masturbation. Dennerstein and colleagues[20] found no relationship between hormone replacement in females and desire for sex, enjoyment of sex, ability to reach orgasm or ease of vaginal lubrication. They did find, however, as did Huffman,[45] a significant relationship between preoperative anxiety concerning possible deterioration of sexual performance and postoperative loss of desire and increased dyspareunia substantiating previous studies of the effectiveness of self-fulfilling prophesies. Estrogen therapy was not effective against the decreased libido.

Munday and Cox[72] and Utian[94] in separate studies found no correlation between sexual outcome and conservation or destruction of ovarian function.

As with menopausal sequelae, an ongoing, active sexual life seems more prognostic of effective sexual function than is the presence of functional ovaries. In some cases, however, estrogen lack can result in a thinning of the vaginal skin leading to bleeding with intercourse, susceptibility to vaginal infections and diminished vaginal lubrication.

Sexual Counseling

The woman who anticipates possible deterioration of sexual functioning warrants special attention. Intense, skilled counseling and at times psychotherapy—time permitting—will need to be undertaken and continued postoperatively.

Besides the general concepts of counseling already outlined, the proscriptions, timing and types of sexual activity are similar to those following a hysterectomy.

When there are complaints of dyspareunia or dryness of the vagina, a pelvic examination is in order to diagnose the presence or absence of an organic etiology. A pale, easily bruised vaginal skin with loss of rugosity, a dry appearance or superadded vaginitis, signs of an estrogen deficient state, can explain the sexual dysfunction. An estrogen index of the desquamated vaginal cells (by Pap smear), confirms the diagnosis. An estrogen foam or cream used intravaginally every other day is usually sufficient to improve the situation. If not, oral estrogen, when there are no medical contraindications, will be effective.

Preparations—Premarin 0.625 mg. daily for 3 weeks followed, if the uterus is present, by Provera 10 mg. twice a day for 5 days is the usual regimen. Premarin may be substituted by an equivalent dose of a synthetic estrogen (Table 1). Progestin is prescribed cyclically to prevent the possibility of hyperplastic changes of the endometrium from long-term exposure to unopposed estrogen. If the use of estrogen is contraindicated, KY jelly may be used as a lubricant. Petroleum jelly is a poor choice. If placed over the urethral meatus, it may result in its blockage since the jelly is not water-soluble. Needless to say, alcohol-based topical creams or lotions are irritating and injurious to vaginal and vulval skin and should not be recommended. If even this brings no relief to the woman, counseling of the couple on other techniques of sexual activity not requiring vaginal intromission will be necessary. This can prove quite satisfactory to maintain sexual satisfaction if there is no deep-seated intrapsychic or relationship pathology.

TABLE 1. COMPARATIVE PHYSIOLOGIC DOSES OF COMMON ESTROGEN PREPARATIONS

Estrogen	Dose (mg)
Ethinyl estradiol	0.02
Diethylstilbestrol	0.25
Conjugated estrogens	0.625
Estrone	1.25

(From J.W. Roddie, Jr., Clin. Obstet. Gynec., Vol. 20, Dec. 1977, p. 909.)

TUBAL LIGATION

"Tubal ligation" is often an inaccurate description of these procedures, since most of them involve removal or destruction of a segment of each fallopian tube rather than a simple ligation.

The tubal ligation may be performed very shortly after childbirth—post-partum tubal ligation—or thereafter, "interval" procedure. The procedure may be performed through an incision in the lower abdomen or through the vagina. A laparoscopic sterilization utilizes the laparoscope through a 1 cm. subumbilical incision. A segment of each tube is cauterized. Newer techniques utilize clips, rings and bands and some may be reversible.

Misconceptions

Often women believe that when need be the ligatures can be untied, thus renewing fertility. At the other end of the spectrum are women who express continuing anxiety over the "ligatures coming loose." There are fears about the effects on menstruation and sexual feelings, and concern over the fate of ova produced after the procedure.

Some women do not have the ability to recognize the uncertainty of the future holding an event such as divorce, death of an only child, or rejection of the belief in zero population. The physician needs to alert the patient to this.

Psychiatric and Functional Sequelae

Some psychiatric sequelae are the result of the loss of fertility itself. The results may be the same as those mentioned for hysterectomy, but are usually found to a lesser degree because it is easier to mobilize defenses. Barglow et al. stated in their report[7] that tubal ligation is a less extensive procedure, and less well understood by patients. There is less drastic change in the body image with no noticeable effect on menstruation and hence women do not have to accept the loss of the reproductive capacity immediately with such finality.

Data regarding menstrual difficulties following the procedure are conflicting. While several retrospective studies indicate a higher incidence of menorrhagia after sterilization, Kasonde and Bonnar[50] in a prospective study report no significant difference in menstrual blood loss.

Campenella and Wolff's report[13] on the incidence of menstrual difficulties which were of a mild nature conflicts with the above data. Menometrorrhagia and dysmenorrhea occurred in 25 per cent of older women and in 65 per cent of women in the younger age group, especially in those women who had had difficulty with contraceptive techniques, or a limited understanding of the surgical procedure or doubted its permanence. This is corroborated by Moore,[71] and Barnes and Zuspan.[8] Barnes and Zuspan, and Moore in separate studies also found that those women who selected sterilization themselves were more likely to be satisfied with it than the women who had tubal ligation suggested to them for medical reasons. Haynes and Wolfe[40] feel that the psychologic responses are dependent upon the doctor-patient relationship and the availability of suitable counseling services. All of this points to the importance of adequate *preoperative counseling complete with explanations of the procedure*. It also demonstrates the group at highest risk and hence worthy of close attention. Neil and co-workers[73] report that the higher frequency of problems with the laparoscopic group may be a result of increased tissue destruction with the resultant compromise of blood supply. In a letter to the editors of *Lancet*, McCann and Kessel[59] disputed this view concerning laparoscopic sterilization, citing their findings of increased and decreased menstrual loss as indicative of causative factors other than the sterilization procedure itself.

Effects on Sexual Functioning

For some women, tubal ligation results in an increased capacity to enjoy sex, and it has been demonstrated in some studies that an increase in libido is more likely for this group than for those who have undergone hysterectomy.

We have also seen cases where the spouse was not consulted or did not approve and the procedure was interpreted by him as punishment or a challenge to his manly powers. Sterilization can make dysfunctional or compromised relationships worse or serve as a focus for further division. This can be prevented in some cases by our assumption that this is a major decision which would best be served by the partner's involvement preoperatively. In Khorana and Vyas' report on women undergoing voluntary sterilization by salpingectomy,[51] 1 per cent resumed sex one month after their operation, 70 per cent between 1½ and 4½ months, 29 per cent remained abstinent due to fears of complications, doubts of the success of the operation, lack of desire, and physical complaints. There was a change in total coital frequency, with 45 per cent having a decrease in frequency, 19 per cent the same and 6 per cent an increase in frequency. Sexual problems were manifested in 6 per cent of the women becoming nonorgasmic and 8 per cent frigid. Nevertheless, 92 per cent were satisfied with the operation while 7 per cent regretted the operation.[51]

Sexual Counseling

Special attention needs to be given to the high-risk group—young women with small families and those to whom tubal ligation was suggested. Partner involvement in a steady relationship is desirable to prevent mental discord and augment emotional support for the woman.

Sexual activity may be resumed once the abdominal incision has healed and the physical activity of sexual relations is not uncomfortable. While women are commonly advised to abstain for four to six weeks, there are no data to substantiate this advice. It is best to utilize the couples' needs and their ability to cooperate and recognize limitations when determining the timing for resumption of intercourse.

DILATATION AND CURETTAGE

The D & C (dilatation and curettage) of the uterus involves the dilatation of the cervical canal and a scraping-off of the superficial layers of the endometrium. This is undertaken for diagnostic and therapeutic purposes.

Misconceptions

Women invest this procedure with the power to increase fertility, cleanse internal organs and even cure certain sexual and menstrual problems.

Anatomical, Psychiatric and Functional Sequelae

Some women can become disappointed when the procedure does not eliminate all of their genitally connected problems. Others manifest a great deal of relief traceable to the concept of cleansing. Ordinarily this procedure is not associated with any significant emotional stress.

There are no profound organic changes except for the presence of a raw endometrial surface which usually completely regenerates within three weeks of the procedure. We are unable to obtain data as to any effects on sexual functioning. We have found virtually none.

Sexual Counseling

A cessation of genital bleeding following the procedure signifies complete regeneration of the endometrium. In our experience this usually takes three weeks. Penile entry of the vagina after this period of time should pose no appreciable threat of ascending infection, although no objective data are available.

Once again, counseling should be specific and explanations given to ensure better compliance.

SURGICAL PROCEDURES ON THE VULVA AND VAGINA

In our experience, common procedures such as episiotomy (an incision on the perineum for childbirth), incision or excision of a Bartholin abscess or cyst, biopsy of the vulva are not associated with appreciable long-term sexual sequelae. Occasionally the procedure may act as an excuse against unpleasant or undesired sexual relations.

Misconceptions

Occasionally there are unrealistic assumptions of the effect of the procedure on sexual functioning. In the case of vaginoplasty—a procedure to remove redundant vaginal tissue, raise a dropped bladder and repair a scarred, relaxed perineum—fulfilling the expectations of cosmetic benefits and enhanced functioning is often beyond the physician's capabilities, regardless of his expertise.

Some women interpret the illness and surgical correction as punishments for past indiscretions.

Anatomical, Psychiatric and Functional Sequelae

There is a paucity of documented information available to date. In our experience, the surgical procedure usually relieves unpleasant symptoms and discomfort without any profound psychiatric or functional changes. Occasionally zealous suturing of the perineal muscles to improve perineal tone and introitus size may prove to cause discomfort at penile entry for an extended period of time.

Most gynecologists do in fact take the precaution of judging the size of the introitus for adequacy prior to repair of the perineum.

Effects on Sexual Functioning

Since most gynecologists advise a conservative six weeks before return to sexual activity, most couples do so gingerly and no significant negative sequelae are observed. In fact, many younger patients who have undergone perineoplasty are most pleased by the newfound feeling of snugness of the vagina.

Sexual Counseling

Counseling that encourages intimacy and lessens the risk of infection and pain is adequate for most of the procedures.

In the case of vaginoplasty we have not been impressed by the objective data available, but some things seem clear. Early resumption of sexual intercourse assures dilatation and pliability of vaginal tissues. In pursuit of the earliest introduction of stretching, the best yardstick is the healing process itself, which should be used as the determining factor. The level of the healing process should be assessed by the gynecologist by the sixth postoperative week. When lifting the proscription of sexual intercourse, it is necessary to counsel about position and depth of thrusting. A set of specific suggestions on techniques needs to be undertaken.

In the case of vaginoplasty for stress incontinence, uterine descensus, or cystorectocele, it is beneficial to teach and prescribe Kegel's exercises to improve muscle tone. Intercourse is the method of choice for dilatation unless medically contraindicated or a partner is unavailable. In those cases where there is no current partner or the penis appears too large for the vagina, dilators of gradually increasing diameter can be utilized by the patient. In the hands of a sensitive partner, the dilators can serve as a useful tool toward the reintroduction of sexual intercourse.

GYNECOLOGIC PROCEDURES FOR MALIGNANCY

Depending upon the organ involved, women who are treated surgically for malignancy of the reproductive tract may have the uterus, tubes, ovaries, upper portion of the vagina, bladder, rectum, clitoris, vulva, or vagina removed. In most instances during the preoperative and immediate postoperative phases, the threat to life is so real that concern over sexual function is usually drawn into the background by the woman and her partner. It is not until much later when the threat seems more remote that the focus begins to shift to functional capabilities.

Misconceptions

Often the disease is looked upon as a punishment for known and unknown "sins." We have witnessed more than one patient offer an unrelenting God her sex life in exchange for survival.

Loss of sexuality and desirability as a sexual partner are late concerns. Many partners have a conscious or unconscious dread of somehow contracting the disease.

Anatomical, Psychiatric and Functional Sequelae

There is a high correlation of these procedures with depression. Some patients feel they are no longer women. For a few, the response is relief. These are major procedures which radically change the woman physically resulting in far-reaching emotional sequelae. A woman's lowered self-esteem and compromised self-image result in a skewed self-perception. If her partner is insecure regarding his self-worth and capacity to express himself as a man, feels guilty as though having caused the problem, or fears catching the disease, there can be avoidance of intimate interaction—both sexual and social. The questions, concerns and fears of both partners can be serious and extensive whenever the procedure is radical. Anytime there is a fear of death added to the equation, the responses have an even greater propensity for distortion. There is such a variety of psychological presets and emotional responses, that a description of the possibilities defies our limited scope. What seems crucial in this regard is the *willingness to pay attention to the specific feelings of our patients,* with our responses being tailored to their specific needs and questions.

The anatomical and functional sequelae depend upon the organs removed. Huffman has reported on three cases of clitoridectomy. He found no effect on orgasm, coitus or sexual desire.[45]

The process of healing is sometimes excessively long, especially for extensive procedures such as pelvic exenteration or when complications such as infection, bleeding, bladder or ureteric injury ensue.

Since the labia are removed at vulvectomy, the perineum may be scarred and lose its normal physical appearance. In the sexually active woman, this can have profound effects on self-image, sense of desirability and confidence in sexual interactions.

Effects on Sexual Functioning

With procedures which are disfiguring or entail the loss of sexually functional organs such as the vagina, the possibility of affecting sexual functioning is profound. The presence of urine and colostomy bags is not conducive to sexual comfort (to put it mildly).

In a strong supportive relationship, many of these obstacles may be overcome, underscoring the value of involvement of a caring and concerned partner.

Sexual Counseling

The emotional reactions of a woman who has undergone vulvectomy need not be stressed. She is aware and concerned about her disfigurement and physical handicaps. The questions, concerns, and fantasies of the patient and her partner are of paramount importance pre- and postoperatively. Open communication must be encouraged between doctor and patient as well as the partner from the outset. It is even more important with this procedure than with most others to *plan for sexual adequacy preoperatively.* Sexual adequacy needs to be as important a concern for the gynecologist in regard to choice of surgical procedure as are the size of the patient, the nature of the disease, and possible risks to the patient based upon age and parity.

The treatment of uterine cancer either surgically or by radiation may have profound effects on sexual activity. The removal of the upper third of the vagina and postoperative fibrosis may result in considerable reduction in the functional length of the vagina. Resumption of regular coitus will gradually stretch the vagina while the use of positions requiring less vaginal depth (e.g., side-to-side) will enable the couple to function in a sexually satisfying manner. In most cases three months is an appropriate waiting time to allow for complete healing. Anxiety related to coitus may be based on the assumption that sex may have caused the disease, resulting in loss of libido of both partners for fear of contracting the disease from their partner. This interferes much more with vaginal function than does radical surgery! Lubrication, lengthening and expansion of the vagina during sexual activity are rarely possible after a full course of radiotherapy which produces serious distortion of the lower genital tract in over 80 per cent of the patients.[3]

CONCLUSION

As we have pointed out, gynecologic surgery is an emotion-laden area for women. Psychological investment in genital, sexual and reproductive organs is heavy. It is incumbent upon the physician to allow the patient to confront and verbalize her feelings, fears, questions, concerns and fantasies about the procedures or outcomes. A serious consideration of the patient as a sexual being preoperatively will enable the physician to plan for and aid a good sexual outcome post-surgically. An incorporated partner can be a very effective therapeutic ally in maximizing a good physiologic and psychologic result. The readiness to provide a comfortable, approachable, willing, listening ear, coupled with individualized education, advice, and support can result in fewer post-surgical complications, dissatisfactions, or discomfort. *Elevating sexuality to the level of importance for the gynecologist that it has for his patients* is an important step toward the treatment of patients as whole people rather than as bodies with diseased parts of which the physician is responsible for only a segment. The extra minutes spent with the woman who has placed her life in our hands can benefit her for years. Consideration of sexual adequacy is her right and our responsibility.

BIBLIOGRAPHY

1. Abeles, M.M. Postoperative psychoses. Am. J. Psychiat. 94:1187–1203, 1938.
2. Ackner, L.B. Emotional aspects of hysterectomy. A follow-up study of fifty patients under the age of 40. Adv. Psychosomat. Med. (Basel) 1:248–252, 1960.
3. Amias, A.G. Sexual life after gynaecological operation—I. Brit. Med. J. 2:608–609, 1974.
4. Andreoli, C. Corpus luteum activity after hysterectomy in women. Acta Endocr. 50:65–69, 1965.
5. Andrew, J.M. Recovery from surgery, with and without preparatory instruction, for three coping styles. J. Personality Soc. Psychol. 15:596–602, 1970.
6. Barglow, P. Pseudocyesis and psychiatric sequelae of sterilization. Arch. Gen. Psychiat. 1:571–580, 1964.
7. Barglow, P., Gunter, M.A. et al. Hysterectomy and tubal ligation: A psychiatric comparison. Obstet. Gynecol. 25:520–527, 1965.
8. Barnes, A.C. and Zuspan, F.P. Am. J. Obstet. Gynaecol. 75:65–71, 1958.
9. Barker, M.G. Psychiatric illness after hysterectomy. Brit. Med. J. 2:91–95, 1968.
10. Benedek, T. Psychosexual Functions in Women. New York, The Ronald Press, 1952.
11. Benedict, R. Psychiatry 1:161, 1938.
12. Bragg, R.L. Risk of admission to mental hospital following hysterectomy or cholecystectomy. Am. J. Public Health 55:1403–1410, 1965.
13. Campenella, R. and Wolff, J.R. Emotional reaction to sterilization. Obstet. J. 45:332–344, 1971.
14. Chafetz, M.E. Hysterectomy and castration-emotional lookalike. Medical Insight 3:38–44, 1971.
15. Chakravarti, S., Collins, W.P. et al. Endocrine changes and symptomatology after oophorectomy in premenopausal women. Brit. J. Obstet. Gynaecol. 84:769–75, 1977.
16. Chynoweth, R. Psychological complications of hysterectomy. Austr. New Zealand J. Psychiat. 7:102–104, 1973.
17. Cobb, S. and McDermott, N.T. Post-operative psychosis. Med. Clin. N. Amer. 22:569–576, 1938.
18. Dalton, K. Discussion on the aftermath of hysterectomy and oophorectomy. In section of general practice, Proc. Roy. Soc. Med. 50:415–418, 1957.
19. Decker, W.H. and Schwartzman, E. Sexual function following treatment for carcinoma of the cervix. Amer. J. Obstet. Gynec. 83:401, 1962.
20. Dennerstein, L., Wood, C. and Burrows, G.D. Sexual response following hysterectomy and oophorectomy. Obstet. Gynecol. 49:92–96, 1977.
21. Dennerstein, L., Wood, C. and Burrows, G.D. Sexual dysfunction following hysterectomy. Austral. Family Physician 6:May 1977.
22. D'Escopo, D.A. Hysterectomy when the uterus is grossly normal. Am. J. Obstet. Gynecol. 83:113–122, 1962.
23. Deutsch, H. Some psychoanalytic observations in surgery. Psychosomat. Med. 4:105–115, 1942.

24. Dodds, D.T., Potgieter, C.C. et al. The physical and emotional results of hysterectomy: A review of 162 cases. S. Afr. Med. J. 35:53–54, 1962.
25. Donahue, V.C. On elective hysterectomy: Pro and con. New Eng. J. Med.:264–295, 1976.
26. Douglas, G. Emotional problems associated with hysterectomies. J. Am. Osteopath. Assoc. 7:1345–1346, 1971.
27. Drellich, M.G. and Bieber, I. The psychologic importance of the uterus and its functions. J. Nerv. Ment. Dis. 116:322–336, 1958.
28. Drellich, M.G., Bieber, I. and Sutherland, A.M. The psychological impact of cancer and cancer surgery. VI. Adaptation to hysterectomy. Cancer 9:1120–1126, 1956.
29. Ebaugh, F.G. The psychiatrist in relation to surgery. Surg. Gynec. Obstet. 69:372–376, 1939.
30. Egbert, L.D., Batti, G.W. et al. Reduction of postoperative pain by encouragement and instruction of patients. New Eng. J. Med., 825–827, 1964.
31. Ellison, R.M. Psychiatric complications following sterilization of women. Med. J. Austral. 2:625–628, 1964.
32. Ewalt, J.R. Psychiatric preparation of the surgical patient. Mod. Hosp. 53:62–63, 1939.
33. Field, R.J. and Field, R.J., Jr. Effect of hysterectomy on young women. Miss. Doctor 36:31–32, 1958.
34. Ford, C.S. and Beach, F.A. Patterns of sexual behavior. New York, Harper and Row, 1951.
35. Frasier, S.D. and New, M.I. Variation in pituitary-gonadal function in adolescent male homosexuals and heterosexuals. J. Clin. Endocr. Metab. 30:796–801, 1974.
36. Gallo, D. Implications sicologicas relacionadas con histerectomia. Ginec. Obstet. Mexico 26:437–444, 1969.
37. Green, R.L. The emotional aspects of hysterectomy. South. Med. J. 66:442–444, 1973.
38. Golub, L.J. Amer. J. Obstet. Gynec. 66:169, 1953.
39. Hampton, P.T. and Tarnasky, W.G. Hysterectomy and tubal ligation: A comparison of the psychological aftermath. Am. J. Obstet. Gynecol. 119:949–952, 1974.
40. Haynes, D.M. and Wolfe, A.M. Am. J. Obstet. Gynecol. 106:1044–1053, 1970.
41. Henker, F.O. Female genital surgery and mental illness. South. Med. J. 57:746–749, 1964.
42. Hollender, M.C. A study of patients admitted to a general hospital after pelvic operation. Am. J. Obstet. Gynecol. 79:498–503, 1960.
43. Hollender, M.C. Hysterectomy and feelings of femininity. Med. Aspects Hum. Sexuality 6–15, 1969.
44. Horak, J. Sexuologicko-gyneckologicke problemy nasich zen po Abdominalnich Hysterecktomiich a Supravaginalnich Amputachich Delozniho tela. C.S. Gynekologie 26:378–382, 1961.
45. Huffman, J.W. The effect of gynecologic surgery on sexual relations. Amer. J. Obstet. Gynecol. 59:915–917, 1959.

46. Jacobs, W.M., Daily, H.I. and Wills, S.H. The effect of hysterectomy on young women. Surg. Gynec. Obstet. 104:107–309, 1957.

47. Johnson, J.E., Leventhal, H. and Dabbs, J.M., Jr. Contribution to emotional and instrumental response processes in adaptation to surgery. J. Pers. Soc. Psychol. 20:55–64, 1972.

48. Judd, H.L., Judd, G.E. et al. Endocrine function of the post-menopausal ovary: Concentration of androgens and estrogens in ovarian and peripheral vein blood. J. Clin. Endocr. Metab. 39:1020–1024, 1974.

49. Judd, H.L. Clin. Obstet. Gynec. 19:775–788, 1976.

50. Kasonde, J.M. and Bonnar, J. Effect of sterilization on menstrual blood loss. Brit. J. Obstet. Gynaecol. 83:572–575, 1976.

51. Khorana, A.B. and Vyas, A.A. Psychological complications in women undergoing voluntary sterilization by salpingectomy. Brit. J. Psychiat. 127:67–70, 1975.

52. Knutsen, K. The climacteric following supravaginal hysterectomy. Acta Obstet. Gynec. Scand. 32:9–24, 1951.

53. Kroger, W.S. Hysterectomy: Psychosomatic factors of the preoperative and postoperative aspects of management. In Kroger, W.S. (Ed.) Psychosomatic obstetrics, Gynecology and Endocrinology. Springfield, Charles C Thomas, 1962.

54. Letter: Sexual life after gynaecological operations. Brit. Med. J. 3:543, Aug. 30, 1973.

55. Levinson, C.J. Hysterectomy complications. Clin. Obstet. Gynecol. 15:802–26, 72.

56. Lindemann, E. Hysteria as a problem in a general hospital. Med. Clin. N. Amer. 22:592–605, 1938.

57. Lindgren, H.C. An Introduction to Social Psychology (2nd Ed.) John Wiley and Sons, 1973, pp. 277–282.

58. Lu, T. and Chun, D.J. Obst. Gynaecol. Brit. Commonwealth, 74:875–880, 1967.

59. McCann, M.F. and Kessel, E. Late effects of female sterilization (Letter). Lancet 1:37–38, Jan. 8, 1978.

60. McKinley, S.M. and Jeffreys, M. Brit. J. Preventive Soc. Med. 28:108, 1974.

61. Masters, W. and Johnson, V. Human Sexual Inadequacy. Boston, Little, Brown and Co., 1970, p. 286.

62. Meikle, S., Brody, H. and Pysh, F. An investigation into the psychological effects of hysterectomy. J. Nerv. Ment. Dis. 164:36–41, 1977.

63. Melody, G.F. Depressive reactions following hysterectomy, Am. J. Obstet. Gynec. 83:410–413, 1962.

64. Menzer, D., Morris, T. et al. Patterns of emotional recovery from hysterectomy. Psychosomat. Med. 5:379–388, 1957.

65. Meyers, T.J. Psychological effects of gynecic surgery. Pacific Med. Surg. 73:429–432, 1965.

66. Miller, H.H. Acute psychoses following surgical procedures. Brit. Med. J. 1:558–559, 1939.

67. Mills, W.G. Depression after hysterectomy. Lancet 2:672, 1973.

68. Money, J. Components of eroticism in man: The hormones in relation to sexual morphology and sexual desire. J. Nerv. Ment. Dis. 132:239–248, 1961.

69. Monti, P.M., Brown, W.A. and Corriveau, D.P. Testosterone and components of aggressive and sexual behavior in man. Am. J. Psychiat. 136:692, 1977.

70. Moore, J.T. and Tolley, D.H. Depression following hysterectomy, Psychosomat. 17:86–89, 1976.

71. Moore, D.W. Am. J. Obstet. Gynecol. 101:350–351, 1968.

72. Munday, R.N. and Cox, L.W. Med. J. Austral. 2:759–763, 1967.

73. Neil, J.R., Hammond, G.T. et al. Late complications of sterilization by laproscopy and tubal ligation. A controlled study. Lancet 2:699–700, 1975.

74. Newton, N. and Baron, E. Reactions of Hysterectomy: Fact or Fiction? Primary Care, pp. 781–801. Philadelphia, W.B. Saunders, 1976.

75. Patterson, R.M. and Craig, J.B. Misconceptions concerning the psychological effects of hysterectomy. Am. J. Obstet. Gynecol. 85:104–111, 1973.

76. Patterson, R.M., Craig, J.B. et al. Social and medical characteristics of hysterectomized and nonhysterectomized psychiatric patients. Obstet. Gynec. 15:209–216, 1960.

77. Polivy, J. Psychological reactions to hysterectomy: A critical review. Am. J. Obstet. Gynecol. 118:417–426, 1974.

78. Raphael, B. The crisis of hysterectomy. Austral. New Zeal. J. Psychiat. 6:106–115, 1972.

79. Reycraft, J.L. Amer. J. Obstet. Gynecol. 69:543, 1955.

80. Richards, D.H. A post-hysterectomy syndrome. Lancet 1:983–985, 1974.

81. Richards, D.H. Depression after hysterectomy. Lancet 2:430–432, 1973.

82. Rioux, J.E. J. Reprod. Med. 19:329–340, 1977.

83. Rodgers, J. Hysterectomies: A quandary for woman, Los Angeles Times, Sept. 21, 1975.

84. Roeske, N.A. Unpublished data from a study of 21 posthysterectomy women, 1975.

85. Schwyhart, W.R. and Kutner, S.J. A reanalyzing of female reaction to contraceptive sterilization. J. Nerv. Ment. Dis. 156:354–370, 1973.

86. Speert, H. Ann. Surg. 129:468, 1949.

87. Steiner, M. and Aleksandrowicz, D.R. Psychiatric sequelae to gynecological operations. Israel Ann. Psychiat. Related Disciplines 8, 1970.

88. Stengel, E., Zeitlyn, B.B. and Rayner, E.H. Postoperative psychoses. J. Ment. Sci. 104:389, 1958.

89. Stone, S.C., Dickey, R.P. and Mickal, A. The acute effect of hysterectomy on ovarian function. Am. J. Obstet. Gynec. 121:193–197, 1975.

90. Studd, J.W. Brit. J. Obstet. Gynaecol. 84:769–775, 1977.

91. Sutherland, A.M. and Orbach, C.E. Psychological impact of cancer and cancer surgery. II. Depressive reactions associated with surgery for cancer. Cancer 6:958–962, 1953.

92. Sutherland, A.M., Orbach, C.E. et al. Psychological impact of cancer and cancer surgery. I. Adaptation to the dry colostomy. Preliminary report and summary of findings. Cancer 5:857–872, 1952.

93. Thompson, B., Hart, S.A. and Durno, D. J. Biosocial Science 5:71, 1973.

94. Utian, W.H. Effect of hysterectomy, oophorectomy and estrogen therapy in libido. Internat. J. Gynaecol. Obstet. 13:97–100, 1975.

95. Vermuelen, A. J. Clin. Endocr. Metab. 42:267, 1976.

96. Washburne, A.C. and Carns, M.L. Postoperative psychosis. Suggestions for prevention and treatment. J. Nerv. Ment. Dis. 82:508–513, 1935.

97. Wengraf, F. Psycho-neurotic symptoms following hysterectomy. Am. J. Obstet. Gynec. 52:645, 1946.

98. Whitelaw, R.G. J. Obstet. Gynaecol. Brit. Empire 65:917, 1958.

99. Wolf, S.R. Emotional reactions to hysterectomy. Postgrad. Med. 47:156, 1970.

100. Wolfer, J.A. and Davis, C.E. Assessment of surgical patients' pre-operative emotional condition and postoperative welfare. Nurs. Res. 19:402–414, 1970.

101. Wright, R.C. Hysterectomy: Past, present and future. Obstet. Gynecol. 33:560–563, 1969.

102. Youngs, D.D. and Wise, T.N. Changing Perspective on Elective Hysterectomy. Primary Care, pp. 765–779. Philadelphia, W.B. Saunders, 1976.

103. Zeros, S.K. and Papaloucas, A.C. Psychosomatic disturbances following hysterectomy performed at a premenopausal age. Int. Surg. 75:802–804, 1972.

104. Kraemer, H.C., Becker, H.B. et al. Orgasmic frequency and plasma testosterone levels in normal human males. Arch. Sex. Behav. 5:125–132, 1976.

14

Drug Therapy and Sexual Function in the Older Patient

ALEX COMFORT, M.B.

Drugs affect sexual physiology more often and more markedly in older than in younger people because 1) normal erectile physiology changes with age, 2) susceptibility to drug action, especially to autonomic, circulatory and other side effects, increases, and 3) the conditions requiring medication increase in frequency with age. Minor physiological changes, such as a change in the sensation or frequency of ejaculation, which might have escaped notice in youth, are also read by older males in the light of a folklore of declining function with age, and can produce disproportionate psychological effects. The sexual pharmacology of middle and later life results from an interaction of these factors; the task of the prescriber is to understand the normal course of age changes in sexual response and to avoid disturbing function. Since at all ages sexual dysfunction is overwhelmingly psychic in origin, the use of medication to improve function is largely confined to restraining disease conditions (diabetes, arthritis) which actively hinder sexual function, rather than giving drugs which "improve" it. In both cases, reference will be made here chiefly to male functions (erection, ejaculation). Medication unquestionably affects sexual response in women as well as in men, but for cultural reasons, and because of the greater complexity of female sexual physiology, no serious attempt has been made in past literature to document any but the grossest changes. It is virtually certain that drugs are prescribed which interfere with the pattern of orgasm in women, but male-oriented clinicians have not documented them, and patients have not reported them.

It is important to recognize that human sexual function, especially in the male, is *highly idiosyncratic,* both in the interrelation of erectile and ejaculatory functions, and in the response of these to drugs. Medication which produces impotence in one individual may produce non-ejaculation or retrograde ejaculation in another and be without sexual effect in a third, as has been documented in the case of thioridazine (Mellaril).[12] Some of these differences may be attributable to differing metabolism or accessibility of neurotransmissors, to differences in sympathetic-parasympathetic balance, or to central effects of the drugs, but in general idiosyncracy becomes more marked with age. It is likely that drugs similarly affect the incidence and intensity of tumescence, lubrication and orgasm in women. These changes are almost wholly undocumented, as part of the excessive cultural concentration on male sexual physiology, where it is possible, and indeed necessary, to observe the outward and visible signs of an inner and spiritual grace.

Increased libido and erectile performance are relatively rare and equally idiosyncratic effects of medication. While in women androgen administration almost invariably increases libido, some men remain potent and active in the virtual or total absence of testicular androgen; in others androgen may be highly effective in lowering the threshold of excitation, while in yet others it fails to produce any evident result. This simply reflects the fact that there is more than one cause of non-erection, since hypogonadal and so-called "climacteric" impotency respond to testosterone better than impotency which appears to be mainly a learned behavior.[6] The role of androgen in the cycle of male excitation is not known—it is at least as likely that high levels result from, rather than cause, sexual arousal.[13] The overall but irregular decline in cross-sectional androgen levels with increasing age reported by various authors represents not only endogenous reduction, but most probably a reduction in sexual activity imposed by a social "script."[8] One possibly important factor is the fact that in both sexes, fantasy—which in humans is probably the most important single determinant of sexual arousal—is said to decline with age. Whether the sixfold decline in speed of erection observed between ages 20 and 50 is involved with autonomic changes, role-playing, or both, remains to be explored[18]—its importance for function is negligible in sexually educated males.

The overriding importance of social roles, social expectation, socially propagated anxiety, together with the uniqueness of the uses made by man of sexuality, explain why comparative studies on age changes and on hormone effects (e.g., in rats) are not only irrelevant but often actively misleading, and thus have been omitted from this review. The main relevant primate findings would be on the interrelationship between sexuality and dominance in agonic species—old age has not yet been adequately observed in large hedonic apes—because of the uneasy mixture in humans of sexual components drawn from those two moods ("baboonery" and "chimpanism"). The role of the penis as a dominance signal, and erection as both invitation and dominance display, is clearly critical to the Freudian view of human psychosexual development, which is atypical in that males are recognized as competitive when they reach walking age, and the dominance releaser is sited in the genitalia themselves, not in the secondary sexual characters.[5] Part of the instability of the human erectile capacity for stress probably reflects adaptation in favor of the most dominant male, the result brought about in mice by the resorption of fetuses in pregnant females when a less-dominant mate is displaced.[4] It is in the period of middle-age, when status is most threatened, that erectile physiology undergoes the most marked changes.

NORMAL AGE CHANGES

In healthy people of both sexes, sexual activity and capacity for intercourse and orgasm are lifelong. Female response changes little with age—there is no documentation of any slowing of arousal. Changes toward greater or lesser responsiveness after menopause are probably attitudinal, depending on such factors as anxiety over the social image of age and the end of the reproductive role on one hand, and relief at the end of pregnancy risk and contraceptive hassles on the other. In middle-aged women today, resexualization is more common than loss of interest—satisfactory orgasm and coitus quite often persist into the eighth and even the ninth decade when opportunity exists.

The chief change that occurs with normal aging in the male is a slowing of response. Erection takes longer and is less often purely psychic; instead of occurring in response to sexual imagery or a sexual situation, it requires direct stimulation of the penis. Ejaculation is also delayed, and commonly does not occur at every act of intercourse.

The importance of these changes is that they can readily be exaggerated by common medications—and that both the changes themselves and any such exaggeration may be misread by the patient with vicious-circle effects on potency. For men with a relaxed and uncompulsive pattern of sexual expression, the normal age changes are seen as an increase in the capacity for enjoyment, but for men whose stereotype of virility involves hurried response followed by rapid completion of intercourse, they are interpreted as "failure." This may be reported as impotence, and it can lead to genuine impotence through increased anxiety over performance.

It is a help both to the prescriber and to the patient to realize that impotency is not a feature of aging and is never due to chronologic age alone. Sexual dysfunction is in fact extremely common at all ages, and at all ages psychic causes predominate over organic. These include negative attitudes to sexuality generally, performance anxiety and unphysiological notions of what "virility" involves, together with more complicated hostilities and unconsicous factors. Relief of the dysfunction involves correction of these attitudes. While the younger person requires to be disabused of folklore about sex, the older person requires to be disabused of folklore about both sex and aging, and has to contend with a new set of unstabilizing fears and problems. These include heightened performance anxiety due to expectation of failure, misreading of normal physiological changes, loss of self-esteem and partner attractiveness in terms of the culture's prejudice against older people, use of "age" as an excuse to opt out of sexual activity by those who have always found it an anxious business, guilt-disuse-unfamiliarity interactions following bereavement and remarriage ("widower's impotency"), and many similar factors in which folklore regarding sex and aging play a leading part.

At the same time, organic pressures on sexual function do increase with age. They include increased susceptibility of the erectile mechanism to alcohol and other drugs, obesity, diabetes, and conditions such as hypertension or prostatic enlargement in which medical treatment or needlessly radical surgery can upset function. Organic and iatrogenic factors are clearly of importance in assessing medication at any age, and in later life their frequency increases, but even when organic or iatrogenic effects are present, misinformation, anxiety and self-inhibition are usually present as well, and make the difference between mildly impaired and absent function. Sexual dysfunction at any age is treated by withdrawal of physical factors which aggravate it and by counseling. Drugs have little place in its management, save in cases where pain, depression or specific conditions such as diabetes are interfering with libido or autonomic function—the physician can far more often cure dysfunctions by withdrawing drugs which are provoking them. Management of potency problems lies in sexual counseling and in avoidance of iatrogenic interference with function, which increases sharply with age. The old notions of rejuvenation and resexualization, especially with hormones, are almost wholly erroneous.

CHANGES INDUCED BY DRUGS

Changes induced by drugs are superimposed on this normal pattern of change. There are large individual variations which depend both on the physiology and self-confidence of the patient, but males of all ages seem to fall into one of two patterns: those who respond to fatigue, medication, or psychic factors such as unfamiliarity of partner with failure of *erection,* and those who respond to the same factors by failure of *ejaculation.* Erection can be inhibited at any age by a variety of sedatives—the most common contributor to impotence at all ages being *alcohol.* With increased age, small amounts of alcohol can inhibit erection when large amounts formerly did not; in addition, alcohol displays synergy with many other drugs including anticonvulsants and antihistamines. *Ganglionic blocking agents* vary markedly in their effect on sexual physiology. The extreme complexity of erectile physiology[24] and the fact that different mechanisms seem to operate in different people is sufficient to explain this large variation. Many hypotensive agents can affect potency, guanethidine, reserpine and methyldopa commonly, prazosin more rarely. Propranolol does not usually affect potency directly, although this has been reported,[11] but may induce depression with loss of libido. Thiazides do not affect potency, and if problems appear after prolonged treatment, diabetes should be excluded. Among other commonly prescribed drugs, clofibrate can affect both potency and libido—the mechanism is unclear.

A number of drugs act in susceptible individuals to prolong the pre-ejaculatory interval or even suppress ejaculation. These include phenothiazines, tricyclic antidepressants, and monoamine oxidase inhibitors: both imipramine and phenelzine are effective therapeutic agents in "premature ejaculation." In older individuals this effect compounds the normal tendency to later and rarer coital orgasm. Moreover, adrenergic blocking agents may produce not impotency but retrograde ejaculation.[23] In this process semen is projected not down the urethra but into the bladder—it can occur following prostatectomy, in diabetes[2] and spontaneously for unknown reasons—its cultivation "to conserve the semen" is a traditional feat in yoga, so it can evidently be learned as a habit.

Impotency and feminization may naturally follow estrogen therapy for prostatic carcinoma, and impotency alone in the use of antiadrenergic agents.

CLINICAL ASSESSMENT OF DRUG-RESPONSE IN THE MALE

Patients do not always complain of changes in sexual function. Nor do they always analyze the difference between loss of libido, non-erection, non-ejaculation and retrograde ejaculation (though the sexually aware will do so). The most common response to any major interference with sexual function is probably simple noncompliance, which may mystify the physician. This can be avoided if rapport in the discussion of sexuality has been established before medication is ordered. If a few questions concerning sexual function are included in the initial history, the need to instruct the patient to report changes of function in response to medication is avoided (some people will become impotent on aspirin if instructed to monitor their response), and the patient's positive or negative attitude to sexuality and its discussion can be assessed. Repetition of the same questions at each review provides an opportunity for any drug effect to be reported.

In the patient *who complains of loss of function,* taking a proper history is itself part of therapy. In excluding drug-related causes, it is necessary to establish the precise nature of the change in function (loss of interest, non-erection, non-ejaculation, altered ejaculation); to inquire specifically about alcohol consumption; and occasionally to perform the "plastic bag test" (used routinely by British geriatricians for any inexplicable symptom in older persons: the patient is instructed to bring in a single bag *every* medication prescribed, bought over the counter, borrowed from neighbors, which he or she is taking). In any case of sexual dysfunction, whether or not a drug- or disease-related cause is suspected, anxiety will be present, reassurance and information should be given, and an early review appointment set, so that counseling may be instituted if the dysfunction outlives the pharmacologic cause.

Although drug-related dysfunctions in women have not been documented, they will not be documented unless they are sought; thus the same questions should be addressed to female patients so that they may be documented. The only common response to medication acting on the autonomic system which can surface as "sexual dysfunction" in women which is now recognized is urinary incontinence at orgasm in the absence of pelvic floor weakness. Overlubrication in response to estrogen supplements can present as dysfunction in the male. In a couple of approximately the same age, estrogen supplements for periclimacteric symptoms in the woman often coincide with the need for stronger penile stimulation in the man, who may complain that he "has lost sensation" or "feels nothing." This is a common syndrome, but it has not been widely noted in counseling literature.

HORMONE THERAPY IN RELATION TO AGE AND SEXUALITY

Indiscriminate hormone therapy in women extending beyond the immediate period of the menopause, and even the lifelong maintenance of menstrual cycles[26] have been widely promoted in popular literature, and sometimes practiced. The main justifications offered for continued hormone therapy in the absence of cycle irregularity or hot flashes have been maintenance of well-being and sexual function, and the avoidance of eventual senile osteoporosis. Wiser counsels indicate that since one woman in three on continuous or cyclical estrogen therapy will get glandular cystic or adenomatous hyperplasia,[7,21,25] the hazards of the exercise exceed the advantages, although the hyperplasia resolves with progestogen therapy and its incidence is far lower where combined therapy is used to induce endometrial shedding. In view of the fact that even combined therapy involves mandatory sampling of the endometrium at yearly intervals and may obscure malignancy, the supposed cosmetic and sexual effects alone do not justify it. Sexual dysfunction due to failure of lubrication, atrophy and other local genital changes is probably a response less to estrogen deficit than to disuse: there is a strong clinical impression that it rarely occurs in women who remain sexually active, and when it does, local application with monitoring of blood levels is preferable to systemic hormone treatment. It seems likely that the higher levels of sexual activity and expectation and the lower incidence of gynecologic injury from repeated childbirth in the next generation of women reaching menopause will protect sexual function without recourse to estrogen.

HORMONE SUPPLEMENTATION IN MALES

Although androgens can increase libido and the frequency of spontaneous erection in males, this action is irregular (their action on libido in women is in fact far more consistent). Androgen levels do not decrease strikingly with age, nor do blood androgen levels correlate with retention or loss of sexual function. The large and contradictory older literature is confused by the widespread belief in the normality of "senile impotence" and a lack of recognition of psychic and role-playing factors in producing erectile dysfunction. Serious study of the erectile capacity of older males dates from the work of Masters and Johnson.[15] Much of the action of testosterone is on the spinal erectile arc[9] although it also has central effects. It seems clear that although the crude blood androgen level is not a good point of access to function, in view of changes in binding power, androgen deficit is not a major cause of sexual dysfunction in older males.[3,10,16,19,22] Where administered androgen improves sexual function, as it occasionally does, this effect may represent a combination of lowered excitation threshold and increased general well-being. Mesterolone is probably preferable to natural hormones for this purpose,[20] since its use does not inhibit the endogenous production of androgen.[14] Beside lowering the erectile threshold[17] this substance tends to increase or re-initiate spermatogenesis. The trial of androgens in sexual dysfunction of older males involves discounting any physiological action of the hormone against the effects of leading the patient to rely on a pill when attitudinal causes need to be remedied. The results of this trade-off have to be individually assessed, since improvement in the center-stage symptom may be needed to render the attitudinal problem accessible.

It seems probable that while female arousal can be reliably mediated by androgen, the control of male arousal depends on an earlier, probably oligopeptide, neurohormone. Increased libido is consistently seen in males after administration of HCG,[1] when it is administered for infertility. This action probably depends upon FSH or LH or both, or on a specific peptide as yet unidentified, paralleling the arousal seen in animals of both sexes after intraventricular LHRH injection. This group of responses is insufficiently investigated to yield clinical application at present, but the irregular response to androgen in cases of reduced male libido clearly indicates that other mechanisms are involved. To the extent that libidinal decline is not wholly sociogenic it may be integrated with the hypothalamic aging "clock."

SUMMARY

Drug effects on sexual function in the aging are superimposed on existing misconceptions about sexuality and about aging, and on the normal adjustments which occur in sexual physiology with age. They are important because of the added performance anxiety or loss of sexual self-esteem which the culture imposes on the old, the increased need for medication likely to affect autonomic and vascular response, and the increased sensitivity of older persons to drug side effects. Sexual function expressed in intercourse and orgasm is normally lifelong in the absence of disease or social inhibition. The physician should monitor medication to avoid any risk of disturbing this function.

REFERENCES

1. Amelar, R.D. and Dubin, L. J.A.M.A. 237:2423, 1977.
2. A.M.A Editorial. J.A.M.A. 199:661, 1967.
3. Borsch, G. Fortschr. med. 92:222, 1974.
4. Bruce, H.M. and Parkes, A.S. J. Reprod. Fertil. 2:195, 1961.
5. Comfort, A. Lancet 2:107, 1960.
6. Cooper, A.J., Ismail, A.A.A. et al. Brit. Med. J. 3:17, 1970.
7. Ferin, J. and Thomas, K. *In* Aging and Estrogens. Frontiers Hormone Res. 2:134, 1973.
8. Gagnon, J.H. and Simon, W. Sexual Conduct. Chicago, Aldine Press, 1973.
9. Hart, B.L. Science 155:1283, 1967.

10. Kent, J.R. and Agone, A.B. *In* Androgens in Normal and Pathological Conditions (A. Vermeulen, Ed.) Amsterdam, Excerpta Medica Fdn., 1966, pp. 31-35.
11. Knarr, J.W. Ann. Intern. Med. 85:259, 1976.
12. Kotin, J., Wilbert D.E. et al. Amer. J. Psychiat. 133:82, 1976.
13. Kraemer, H.C., Becker, H.B. et al. Arch. Sexual Behav. 5:125, 1976.
14. Ludvik, U. Urologie 9:41, 1970.
15. Masters, W.H. and Johnson, V.E. Human Sexual Inadequacy. Boston, Little Brown, 1970.
16. Papanicolaou, A.D., Adamopoulos, D.A. et al. J. Obstet. Gynec. 77:961, 1970.
17. Schellen, M.C.M. Acta Endocr. (Suppl.) 138:100, 1969.
18. Solnick, R.L. Unpublished data (M.Sc. thesis, Univ. S. California), 1975.
19. Stearns, E.L., Macdonnell, J.A. and Kaufman, B.J. Amer. J. Med. 57:761, 1974.
20. Steinbeck, H. and Neumann, F. Actuelle Gerontol. 8:531, 1974.
21. Sturdee, D.W., Wade-Evans, T. et al. Brit. J. Obstet. Gynec. (In press)
22. Vermeulen, A., Rubens, R. and Verdonck, L.J. Clin. Endocr. Metab. 34:730, 1972.
23. Walden, P. Lancet 1:308, 1969.
24. Weiss, H. Ann. Intern. Med. 76:793, 1972.
25. Whitehead, M.I., McQueen, J. et al. Acta obstet. gynec. Scand. 65:91, 1977.
26. Wilson, R.A. Feminine Forever. London, W.H. Allen, 1966.

15

The Need for Management
of the Psychosexual Aspects
# of Mastectomy

CECILY GREEN, JOANNE E. MANTELL, M.S.S.W., M.S.P.H.

Despite the increasing trend toward humanistic health care, the medical establishment has not given adequate recognition to the various sexual sequelae of a chronic illness such as cancer. The primary modalities of treatment for cancer—surgery, radiation and chemotherapy—have the potential for interfering with patients' sexual expression. Yet the suppressive effects of these routine medical practices are generally not shared with patients and their significant others.[1]

Cancer can have direct physiological consequences on sexual functioning. For example, a colostomy and prostatectomy may cause erectile failure if nervi have been damaged.[2] In the case of spinal cord lesions, there may be a loss of sensation in body parts which have traditionally been a source of sensual pleasure. In addition, the emotional concomitants of cancer can inhibit sexual activity. Some women who have undergone an hysterectomy become sexually unresponsive because surgery is perceived as a symbolic castration, the loss of repro-

An earlier version of this text was presented at the 105th annual meeting of the American Public Health Association, Washington, D.C., 1977.

duction equated with defeminization or asexuality.[3] Changes in the outward appearance of the body can also impair sexual functioning. The gross distortions resulting from certain maxillofacial reconstructive procedures may limit cancer patients' oral sexual expression as well as cause others to react adversely. Poor hygiene of artificial stomas can create barriers to social and physical intimacy.

A mutilating surgical procedure such as mastectomy provides an excellent example of the need for management of the psychosexual repercussions of cancer. Women need to be concerned not only with the physical adjustments, but with the role surgery plays in inducing psychogenic sexual dysfunction. Our culture's preoccupation with the breast as a symbol of femininity is largely responsible for increasing a mastectomee's vulnerability toward sexual maladjustment. A woman's response to this trauma is influenced by components of her social environment since her attitudes and behavior are products of her perception of and interaction with her significant others.

SEXUAL STEREOTYPES IN OUR CULTURE

Our prevailing cultural obsession with appearance as reflected by our media idolization of youthfulness and beautiful bodies can have damaging consequences for the woman without an intact body. The stigmatizing effect of mastectomy places a psychological burden on women with such disfigurement because of aesthetic aversion to physical unattractiveness. In addition, the inequality of sex-role proscriptions contributes to the maintenance and reinforcement of this conception of beauty. While a male's status attainment depends largely on achievement, a woman's social worth is all too often predicated on physical and sexual appeal. Minimal social import is assigned to a man's physical attributes. This double standard is most oppressive to women and depreciates the value of the feminine role. The cumulative effect of these social requisites is damaging to all women's self-concept, but particularly devastating to the mastectomee.

Cultural emphasis on breasts is also reflected in the increased requests for reconstructive surgery following mastectomy. Despite the endowment of a reconstituted breast, which creates an improved physical appearance, there is no assurance that this cosmetic procedure will effect positive psychological results.[4] Rather, a distorted perception of body-image and feelings of inadequacy often remain. Nevertheless, for some women, plastic surgery is a prerequisite for reducing emotional distress and bolstering self-concept.

Women who have undergone mastectomy need to reconcile not only the discrepancy between cultural expectations and their disfigurement, but also deal with their perceived loss of both femininity and sexual desirability. Self-concept and body-image, which are essential components of sexuality, are shaped not only by cultural expectations but also by the internalization and the enactment of others' perceptions and attitudes. The mutilating effect of a breast amputation can be viewed as a damaging blow to self-esteem. Consequently, feelings of anxiety and social unacceptability may result. In addition, if not properly intercepted, the incongruency between actual and ideal body-image can lead to impaired social and sexual relationships.

EFFECTS ON THE UNPARTNERED WOMAN

The woman alone, either single, divorced or widowed, is confronted with unique problems after mastectomy. Following the trauma of dealing with the shock of diagnosis and the decision to proceed with what is hoped will be life-saving albeit mutilating surgery, she is left to adjust to her altered body-image without the support of a committed and caring partner. Women who desire an active sex life may find that after surgery, anticipation of sexual intimacy provokes intense anxiety. Although this feeling usually dissipates with time, some unattached women withdraw totally from male relationships. In extreme cases, such avoidance may lead to social isolation. Other women, fearful that future lovers will not be available, may become preoccupied with defying this potential consequence by resorting to sexual promiscuity.

The following case examples illustrate some of the special problems that the unattached mastectomee may need to face:*

> Case 1. A single, 24-year-old woman, with a history of two long-term relationships, was rejected by her lover at the time of mastectomy. He recoiled in horror at viewing her surgical site and subsequently terminated the relationship because he was no longer "turned on." After months of mourning the loss of her partner, the woman felt socially uncomfortable relating to appropriately eligible men. Eventually the only males with whom she could be secure, either socially or professionally, were significantly younger or older.

> Case 2. A divorced, 48-year-old attractive woman, unable to adjust fully to being deserted by her husband, had just begun attempts to meet eligible men when she learned she had breast cancer. After recovering from surgery, she began to dress provocatively and travel from bar to bar, flirting outrageously with men. Although she did not drink and had not

---

*All case descriptions are derived from the authors' clinical practice.

previously frequented such places, she now had the need for constant validation of her sexual desirability and attractiveness without risking involvement in a stable relationship.

Every unattached woman wrestles with the problem of when and how to disclose her body alteration to a prospective partner. Those women who have told their friends and co-workers that they have had a mastectomy will find that prior to the social introduction, most prospective partners have been informed of the mastectomy. The practice gleaned from being candid with friends and acquaintances often facilitates disclosure of this information to new acquaintances. Dialogue between the woman and a new partner before their first intimate encounter can help both parties cope with their physical and emotional reactions to the sight of the missing breast. Consequently, when the surgery site is actually viewed, shock and aversion may be reduced.

EFFECTS ON THE ADOLESCENT DAUGHTER

Pressures of adolescence are intensified for the girl who must consider the possible loss of her breasts before she has incorporated them as part of her body-image. Being aware of the genetic predisposition to breast cancer is very painful for both daughter and mother, sometimes causing anger and resentment in the former and guilt feelings in the latter. In addition to culpability for her daughter's future bout with breast cancer, a mother may be envious of her nubile daughter's firm, youthful breasts, a sharp contrast to her one remaining withered breast.

Because the diagnosis of breast cancer is usually followed by rapid hospitalization, the head of operations has little time to prepare for the daily maintenance of the household. The not-yet-mature teenaged daughter may be suddenly thrust into the responsibility for cooking, laundry, housework and chauffering, in addition to the care and nurturing of her younger siblings and father. The ensuing resentment and hostility usually expressed toward her convalescing mother can, if viewed empathetically, provide a constructive outlet for her undisclosed feelings of anger about the fear of her mother's premature death, the threatened loss of her own breast and the oppressive weight of assuming adult responsibility without adequate preparation. As her mother struggles with feelings of defeminization after surgery, the adolescent daughter is without a healthy role model for adult female sexuality. At the same time, the father's unacknowledged acute awareness of his daughter's innocent yet full-blown sexuality and the shame he feels as a result of his sexual arousal is often displayed by irritability and possessiveness. Consequently, there may be explosive conflicts with her father over her dating behavior.

Illustrative of some of these issues are the following case reports:

Case 1. A 53-year-old mother and wife who had metastatic disease at diagnosis suffered a protracted illness and convalescence. When the family's limited resources were almost exhausted, they moved to a tiny 2-bedroom cottage, with the invalid mother occupying one bedroom, the father and 29-year-old ne'er-do-well son the second bedroom, and the 16-year-old daughter, the couch in the living room. The cluttering of the cottage with furniture and sickroom supplies made it impossible for the daughter to entertain her friends at home. Consequently, she spent a lot of time outside the household. As privacy was non-existent, the daughter had to change her clothes in the living room. The father became uncomfortably aroused by the sight of his daughter's seemingly constant state of *déshabille* and expressed his painful sexual tension in jealous rages against her boy friends. The daughter was preoccupied with her sexual tension and had no one with whom to explore the perplexities of being a young girl within an adult body.

Case 2. A 33-year-old mother who had an oophorectomy following her breast surgery experienced a shattered sense of sexual self-esteem. Feelings of asexuality precipitated exclusive attention to the mothering role. She became "super-mom" and took great pride in anticipating every need and desire of both her girls. Consequently, when symptoms of advanced metastatic disease appeared eleven years after surgery, her teenaged daughters were totally unprepared to assume any responsibility for running the household. Bitter fights between the mother and the daughters ensued and precipitated the father, exhausted from being arbitrator, to retreat into a severe depression. The disintegration of the family may have contributed to the mother's poor response to treatment.

The unique problems of the adolescent daughter of the mastectomee may require active professional intervention. Without this help, the ravages of the disease extend beyond the victim's body; whereas with the therapeutic benefits of such efforts, the psychological well-being of not only the breast cancer patient but her most significant others will be improved.

EFFECTS ON THE SEX PARTNER

Partners are often initially apprehensive about the sexual consequences of a mastectomy and require a period of adjustment before accommodating to the woman's altered body contour. Since a woman's self-concept after mastectomy may be modified by a partner's reaction, it is especially important to consider sexual problems from the partner's perspective, regardless of whether the partner is a man or another woman.

Many partners are concerned about their mates' physical and emotional fragility and confused about how to respond to this unusual circumstance. There may also be uncertainty about new expectations.[5] Greater understanding of the mastectomee's tribulations is essential for promoting and maintaining sexual satisfaction in both parties.

Partners may be as distressed as the woman when initially either viewing the incision site, the flat or concave chest, or touching the scarred tissue. A partner is often unable to cope with a mastectomee's distorted body-image until after the shock of the unveiled mutilation. Willingness to look at the scar can represent a turning point in the partner's adjustment to mastectomy.[6] Recognition that the woman no longer has an intact body may facilitate integration of the fantasy and reality of the trauma. In addition, a partner's readiness to express negative feelings about the scar and disfigured body ultimately may foster a positive self-concept in the woman.

There may be reluctance to resume sexual activity after surgery for fear of inflicting unnecessary pain. Some partners refrain from hugging because they are afraid of hurting a woman. Although there is no scientific evidence indicating that breast cancer is a sexually-transmitted disease, the fear of contagion may inhibit such basic physical contact as kissing and caressing.

Some of these common issues can be illustrated by the following examples:

> Case 1. A 45-year-old woman who married when she and her husband were in their teens and virgins, was accustomed to physical displays of affection which were always a prelude to coitus in the missionary position. Metastatic lesions in the pubic and pelvic bones were discovered after her breast removal. Although radiation therapy partially reduced these lesions, male superior coitus was still painful because of residual pain in the pelvic area and radiation burns to the vaginal barrel. All physical contact subsequently ceased to circumvent coping with erotic feelings. Having never practiced manual masturbation, self or mutual, the unrelieved sexual tension became un-

bearable. Ensuing irritability and poor communication contributed to the destruction of their relationship.

Case 2. A 51-year-old married woman had reasonably accommodated to her husband's low level of sexual interest prior to mastectomy. He used the surgery, however, as a fortuitous event, releasing himself from the responsibility of cranking up for intermittent sexual interaction. Consequently, he avoided any physical contact so that his intentions would not be misunderstood. At the same time, the woman's recovery was seriously hampered by her unmet need for physical intimacy.

The potential for a mastectomy to precipitate male sexual dysfunction has yet to be explored by sex researchers.[7] The classic secondary sexual dysfunctions of impotence, ejaculatory inhibition and lack of erotic arousal are experienced by some partners and can by very frightening to the uncommunicative and sexually unsophisticated.[7-9] Situational impotence is often caused by anxiety and/or fatigue, ejaculatory inhibition usually emerges as a result of conflict, and lack of affect ("I don't get turned on") is a common symptom of depression. All of these feelings may be precipitated by the highly stressful event of mastectomy. Sexologists recognize that performance anxiety is self-defeating. Temporary sexual dysfunction and its accompanying distress contributes to escalating the problems of adjustment to crisis, which may in turn reinforce the dysfunction.

Another major area affecting sexual adjustment is that most adults have inadequate knowledge about human sexuality. For the man who believes that physical affection is equated with sex, and therefore penile-vaginal intromission, the trauma of dealing with a partner who suddenly faces an assault to her health, body-image and mortality can be emotionally devastating. Accommodations in lifestyle need to be made from the time of initial diagnosis, through surgery and subsequent treatment, perhaps for many years. Adaptive behavior, particularly in the area of sexual expression, may be required to maintain and improve the premorbid status of the relationship.[10]

It is desirable and sometimes necessary to assemble a vast repertoire of new sexual behaviors, including experimentation with coital positions, additional areas of erotic sensitivity and techniques of manual and oral stimulation. The availability of sensitive, empathetic health professionals for education, counseling and therapy is mandatory. In cases where communication between partners is unwieldy, it would be innovative to use a trained surrogate for the partner, a surrogate preferably who has experienced and coped well with her own mastectomy. Together, they can explore experientially feelings about the physical responses to the mastectomy. In addition, there can be experimentation with new modes of sexual expression. This treatment plan is contingent upon the informed consent of both parties in the primary relationship.

EFFECTS ON THE RELATIONSHIP

A woman's attitude toward herself as a sexual being represents an important yardstick for gauging self-esteem and determining the nature of her interaction with others. The quality of postoperative relationships is often contingent upon the woman's response to her changed body-image which, in turn, will set the tone for others' attitudes and reactions toward her. Consequently, assessment of the psychosexual impact of mastectomy needs to be regarded within the interpersonal context.

Postoperative sexual adjustment seems to be predicated on the general nature of the relationship prior to surgery as well as on the strain of the mastectomy itself.[7,11] Couples who have always been physically affectionate and content with the degree of their intimacy may find that breast cancer and subsequent mastectomy will not adversely affect their relationship. In contrast, couples who lack emotional commitment and sexual compatibility will find that the stresses of mastectomy compound their historical problems. Some may use the mastectomy as a vehicle to lessen their sexual involvement in an already burdensome and unrewarding relationship.[12] In extreme cases, all forms of sexual expression may cease. If the woman cannot cope with her partner's increased inattentiveness, she may seek confirmation of her sexual desirability outside the confines of their relationship. At the same time, the further deterioration of the relationship may drive the partner to act in a similar fashion. Most couples fall into the middle of these extremes.

All couples, however, need to contend with various problems affecting their relationship. The unexpressed rage that some women feel toward their male surgeons is often generalized toward all men, particularly those with whom they share physical intimacy.[7] Consequently, frequency of and satisfaction with sexual relations may temporarily diminish and eventually precipitate a partner's alienation if both parties do not have sufficient opportunity to express these negative feelings.

Fear of rejection can be problematic for both the woman and her partner. A woman's perceived sexual undesirability may facilitate the erection of barriers to physical intimacy. Through subtle and often covert signals, she may tacitly communicate that sexual activity is *verboten*. In response, her partner may become physically inattentive, reinforcing her feelings of rejection. Many of these negative feelings are perpetuated because they stem from assumptions which are rarely verified between the partners.

A partner's collaboration in the woman's care can contribute toward decreasing her feelings of isolation as well as his sense of helplessness. Sharing with her in the decision-making processes before surgery may well enhance their adjustment to the woman's altered body-image.[7] Partners can be encouraged to help the woman change her dressings and massage the affected arm. Stimulation not only helps restore lymphatic circulation, but through the resulting physical contact, can ensure familiarity with the deformity.[8] In addition, women who are reluctant to practice breast self-examination of their incision site and the remaining breast can enlist their partners' support. This sharing of responsibility for her health may relieve each of them of some anxiety. At the same time, his participation can provide somatosensory nurturing that may enhance their desire for physical intimacy.

It is important to remember that a mastectomy may require a new lifestyle, directly affecting the sexual relationship. Women who desire more children are often discouraged from having them because of the increased estrogen production resulting from pregnancy. This imposed limitation conflicts with their need to fulfill the mother role. A mastectomy may require new daily living habits that also alter patterns of sexual interaction. Many partners forego routine breast foreplay, limiting the time of sexual contact to that required for climax. To facilitate comfort while sleeping, some women place a pillow under their surgical site or wear a sleeping bra to compensate for the loss of their balance and body symmetry. A woman who uses a pillow to elevate the lymphedematous ipsilateral extremity may need to switch the side of the bed on which she usually sleeps to avoid shielding herself from her partner. Other women will refrain from wearing décolleté bedclothes and retreat to the anonymity of a granny nightgown. Sexual activity may be initiated in and restricted to the dark.[12] In extreme cases, women who react adversely to the sight of their mutilation will insist on maintaining separate bedrooms. If the woman does not explain the reasons for these changes, the sexual partner may perceive them as evidence of sexual disinterest.

The destructive effects of a mastectomy on the sexual relationship can be highlighted by the following anecdotes:

> Case 1. As a result of uterine cancer at the age of 37 and the breakup of her 12-year-old third marriage, a 53-year-old married woman was very vulnerable to loss. Fibrocystic disease of both breasts was carefully observed by her physician. Her fourth marriage to a man many years her junior was never stable from its inception. The problems in the relationship became exacerbated by the increased risk of impending breast loss. After a prophylactic bilateral mastectomy was recom-

mended, her husband encouraged her to have implants. Post-surgical complications, including tissue necrosis, necessitated four separate implant procedures. Her husband's aversion to the sight of her constantly infected chest wall caused him to withdraw from physical contact. Her verbal condemnation of his behavior as well as his inability to be empathetic to her emotional pain led him to seek physical gratification outside the marital relationship. With the marriage floundering, all aspirations for a hopeful future were shattered.

Case 2. A 32-year-old woman used the experience of her mastectomy as an impetus to personal growth. She continued in graduate school and found the satisfaction in her career that was not present in her marriage. Sexual incompatibility was ignored as they both had other sources for enhancement of their self-esteem. When bony metastasis was diagnosed seven years after mastectomy, her world fell apart. Her fear of death became obsessive, and she became sicker and more depressed. They entered therapy together to work on a reconciliation to the idea of her eventual death. The conjoint therapeutic experience with a co-therapy team engendered new ways of communication. As they increasingly shared their deepest feelings, their vulnerability to each other fused the relationship. As her ability to relax increased, she became orgasmic. Both were delighted with her new-found pleasure. As her disease progressed and her body became more distorted, he found himself increasingly responsive to her sexually. Together they experimented with a variety of physical expressions, each one customized to the limitations of her rapidly declining health. The sexual excitation she experienced was like none she had ever known and competed in quality with the release of orgasm after orgasm. This ability to let go generalized into her entire life; the tenacious struggle to refute her dying dissipated. Her relationship with her mother, sons and close friends took on a new quality. Together, they serenely supported one another throughout the period of her terminal illness. She died appropriately, all business resolved. Consequently, her passing at age 43 instilled a new confidence in each of her survivors.

Assuredly, a couple's lack of communication about their mutual anxieties, misunderstandings and expectations may breed dissatisfaction and create a conspiracy of silence. At the same time, professionals who ignore patients' need for candid discussion about their sexual problems compound their existing interpersonal difficulties. Thus, a double-bind is created, and if not attended to, can perpetuate dysfunctional inter-action. On the other hand, sensitive intervention can improve fragile emotional bonds and strengthen solid ones.[6]

CONCLUSION

Although physicians are generally perceived to have the expertise and competence to deal with sexual problems that arise in their medical practice, there is still widespread resistance to direct confrontation of these issues. In light of diminishing taboos against open discussion of sex and increased understanding of human sexual responses, such avoidance seems to be paradoxical. When viewed within the context of medical training, however, this discrepancy can be better explained. Although schools of medicine, nursing and social work are increasingly offering courses on human sexuality, the acquisition of such informa-tion does not ensure that changes in professional behavior will result. Those clinicians who have not been exposed to the sexual parameters of medical care in their professional training generally lack the sophis-tication and *savoir faire* for this task.[13] In addition, discomfort and anx-iety about their own sexual attitudes and behavior limit the ability of some professionals to communicate with patients.[14] At the same time, patients resist candid communication because of their inability to be articulate and their fear of incurring a negative reaction.

Adherence to the traditional medical model can also account for the viewing of cancer patients' sexual problems as of secondary impor-tance. The myth of the physician's magical curative powers is firmly entrenched in his training.[15] The medical profession's preoccupation with curing disease and prolonging life has tended to obfuscate the im-portance of humanistic care. Neglect of patients' psychological needs is often sanctioned in the name of efficiency. Therefore, it is not surprising that most oncologists devote their energies to implementing cancer con-trol measures. Obviously, this type of therapeutic intervention is essen-tial. Such ritualistic, task-centered activity, however, tends to mask the important psychosexual concomitants of cancer.

Although supportive measures are usually deferred until after the mastectomy, attention to the emerging concerns immediately following diagnosis and prior to surgery is also warranted. Increased sensitivity to the woman's needs at this time may not only facilitate preoperative anxiety reduction, but ease the post-surgical adjustment in cases where mastectomy is the outcome. Because sexual expression is important to health maintenance, greater awareness of iatrogenic sexual dysfunction is required. One way in which health professionals can maintain and enhance the quality of cancer patients' precarious existence is to help them and their partners achieve a satisfying and pleasurable level of sexual adjustment.[11]

The responsibility of the primary care physician is to be sensitive to patient vulnerabilities. Although the physician is at the helm of the treatment team, nurses, psychologists and social workers should be available to assist him with the mastectomee's psychosexual needs. In addition, health professionals can instruct women in experiential exercises aimed at restoring their confidence as sexual beings. A variety of community-based support services can also be tapped. The American Cancer Society's Reach to Recovery program trains women who have effectively adjusted to their mastectomies to serve as role models for women facing the immediate aftermath of surgery. In many communities there has been a proliferation of mastectomee consciousness-raising and self-help groups designed to provide continuing emotional support.

The routinization of medical care leads many professionals to forget that a mastectomy is *not* routine for the woman. Consequently, mastectomees are often immobilized by the threat to their sexual being—a threat that might be reduced were caregivers able to envision such surgery from the *patient's perspective*. If physicians are to become other than technical dispensers of treatment, then they must be sensitized to the psychosexual impact of mastectomy on the life style of the woman and her most significant others.

REFERENCES

1. Jacobson, L. Illness and human sexuality. Nursing Outlook 22:50, 1974.
2. Dlin, B.M., Perlman, A. and Ringold, E. Psychosexual response to ileostomy and colostomy. Am. J. Psychiat. 126:374, 1969.
3. Drellich, M.G. Sex after hysterectomy. Med. Aspects Hum. Sexuality 1:62, 1967.
4. Kolin, I.S., Baker, J.L. and Bartlett, E.S. Psychosexual aspects of mammary augmentation. Med. Aspects Hum. Sexuality 8:88, 1974.
5. Asken, M.J. Psychoemotional aspects of mastectomy: A review of recent literature. Am. J. Psychiat. 132:56, 1975.
6. Grandstaff, N.W. The impact of breast cancer on the family. Frontiers Radiat. Ther Oncol. 11:146, 1976.
7. Wellisch, D.K., Jamison, K. et al. Psychosocial Aspects of Mastectomy: Reactions of the Patient's Spouse. Dept. of Psychiatry, UCLA, Center for the Health Sciences, unpublished paper, 1975.
8. Ervin, C.V. Psychologic adjustment to mastectomy. Med. Aspects Hum. Sexuality 7:42, 1973.
9. Golden, J.S. Sexuality and the Chronically Ill. The Pharos of Alpha Omega Alpha 38:76, 1975.

10. Golden, J.S. How You Can Help Patients with Physical Ailments to a Better Sex Life. Med. Times 104:83, 1976.
11. Bard, M. and Sutherland, A. Adaptation to Radical Mastectomy. *In* The Psychological Impact of Cancer, American Cancer Society (Ed.), 1974, pp. 55-71.
12. Jamison, K., Wellisch, D.K. and Pasnau, R.O. Psychosocial Aspects of Mastectomy: The Woman's Perspective, Dept. Psychiatry, UCLA Center for the Health Sciences, unpublished paper, 1975.
13. Pauly, I.B. and Goldstein, S.G. Physicians' ability to treat sexual problems. Med. Aspects Hum. Sexuality 4:24; 30-33; 38; 40; 45-46; 49, 1970.
14. Golden, J.S. Management of sexual problems by the physician, Obstet. Gynec., 23:471, 1964.
15. Feifel, H. Physicians' Attitudes Toward Death. Paper presented at the 75th Annual Convention of the Amer. Psychol. Assoc., Washington, D.C., Sept., 1967.

16

Reducing Post-Mastectomy Sexual Dysfunction: An Appropriate Role for Social Work

JOANNE E. MANTELL, M.S.S.W., M.S.P.H., CECILY GREEN

Introduction

In the last decade increased public disclosure of personal ordeals with cancer has advanced the development of tertiary modes of cancer prevention. A steady stream of information intended to increase aware-ness and knowledge of cancer has flowed from the medical and lay press. Although interventions have traditionally focused on early detec-tion and treatment, the importance of the psychosocial rehabilitation of cancer patients is being more widely recognized by the medical estab-lishment. This trend may be attributed in part to recent medical ad-vances that prolong the lives of cancer patients as well as to greater consumer demand for humanistic care in our increasingly technological and bureaucratic health care system.

Since cancer is now considered to be a chronic rather than an acute disease with a death trajectory, attention needs to be directed not only to living with the disorder, but to maintaining and enhancing the qual-

An earlier version of this text was presented at the 23rd Annual Program Meeting of the Council on Social Work Education, Phoenix, Arizona, 1977, and at the 1977 Na-tional Association of Social Workers Professional Symposium, San Diego, California.

ity of that life. Death education seminars for professionals and the public have gained widespread popularity. Unfortunately, the sexual concerns of the cancer patient still provoke professional resistance.[1] Despite the era of liberalized attitudes and knowledge about sex, the medical community is generally inattentive to the sexual needs of the chronically ill and disabled. The conservatism of health professionals as well as their reluctance to confront these issues directly may hamper their ability to deal with the sexuality of cancer patients.[2]

Although the consequences of such professional behavior have serious ramifications for all cancer patients, women who have undergone a mastectomy are especially vulnerable because of our culture's preoccupation with the sexual connotation of the breast. To many women, a mastectomy means not only the surgical excision of a breast, but loss of femininity, physical attractiveness and sexual desirability. Not only does a woman need to deal with an altered sense of self, she has to learn to cope differently with her network of supportive relationships.

SCOPE OF THE PROBLEM

In our breast-oriented culture, a psychotraumatic event such as mastectomy has wide-range implications for a woman, including possible reduced sexual capacity. Despite the large number of women who develop breast carcinoma, the extensive literature on breast cancer does not present detailed discussions of the sexual adjustment of mastectomees, let alone consider the problem of partners. The breast has been assigned a cultural significance that is in many respects unrelated to its physiologic functions of lactation and erotic stimulation. The breast is not only idealized, but viewed as the symbol of femininity.

Breast surgery may cause a woman to perceive herself as a social outcast because beauty is currently conceived as a function of physical attractiveness and sex appeal. This cultural orientation also contributes to identity problems by compelling women to focus on their physical flaws rather than on their physical attributes. Any deviation from the fashion model image is likely to be viewed as a defect since a body is measured exclusively from a cosmetic viewpoint.

This attitude is responsible for the proliferation of reconstructive breast surgery following mastectomy. As with other types of cosmetic surgery, the reconstituted physical appearance is not necessarily accompanied by improved self-esteem. Nevertheless, to some women, having a body that more closely matches the ideal can provide a more secure environment in which to explore awakening self-appreciation and rebuild self-image.

Sexuality encompasses not only sexual activity but the woman's eroticized self-image. Sexuality is a unique, dynamic process comprising physiologic and psychologic components as well as the internalization of others' perceptions and attitudes. This means that sexual activities are not limited to lovemaking, rather "it is only because they are embedded in social scripts that the physical acts themselves become possible."[3] Sexuality, therefore, includes the sex act, sex drive, sex roles, gender identity, object choice and patterns of interpersonal communication.

Self-concept, which refers to emotional and bodily awareness and the concomitant enactment of these perceptions, is also linked to sexuality. For example, sex appeal is not only equated with breast size, but with a woman's projection of enjoyment of her body. Body image may determine the quantity and quality of interaction with others. After mastectomy, a woman's behavior is reflective of her response to her changed body image. Even when cases of physical disfigurement have been remedied by cosmetic surgery, psychological consequences may remain.[4] No matter how small or inconspicuous the disfigurement, a woman may perceive herself as handicapped,[5] and thus experience lowered self-esteem. This discrepancy between actual physical appearance and distorted body self-image, in turn, may generate anxiety, undermine self-confidence and interfere with normal social and sexual interactions.

THE PSYCHOSEXUAL WORLD OF THE MASTECTOMEE

Women often perceive surgery as an assault or as a punishment. A woman who knows her chest is concave rather than convex may become so anxiety-ridden that she avoids looking at herself.[6] Dressing and bathing serve as painful reminders of her "asexuality," and may become particularly troublesome if she is surrounded by mirrored walls and ceilings. If not intercepted, the woman's aversion to the sight of her "mutilated" body can seriously impair her sexual relationships.

Pinning a prosthesis to her bra before dressing is another tactic that a mastectomee often uses to avoid looking at herself. In many cases, this is a manifestation of postsurgical depression, and may be largely dependent on the social and sexual value that a woman and her family attribute to physical attractiveness. As one woman on the eve of her biopsy expressed:

> "I attract men who have a quiet, deep love for the full, firm softness of large breasts. I sometimes feel I am just the custodian of them and would personally be letting my friends down if I let anyone cut off one of them."

Some mastectomees are so self-conscious that they develop a breast fixation, constantly looking at and evaluating the shape, size and firmness of other women's breasts in relation to their own loss. Feelings of self-deprecation and self-revulsion may be so strong that sexual relations are conducted only in the dark.[7] Negative body-image and wounded self-esteem often lead to decreased responsibility for health, further compounding medical problems, since many women refuse to examine the postoperative site.

Change itself may be viewed as a threat, particularly in lovemaking activities. Women who are accustomed to using their breasts as an integral part of routine sexual foreplay, rather than as passive recipients of their partner's stimulation, will be acutely conscious of their partners' eliminating this activity and urging immediate coital gratification. Even minor changes can be threatening. For example, a woman with postsurgical lymphedema who uses a pillow to elevate the swollen arm may switch the side of the bed on which she normally sleeps to avoid erecting a barrier between herself and her partner. This may result in physical awkwardness and create unease for both parties.

Women fear most the mastectomy's effect on interpersonal relationships. Physical revulsion and fear of rejection by the partner can interfere with sexual responsiveness,[8] making sex a treatment rather than a treat. Some women who expect to be rejected will use disfigurement as a pretext to avoid social relationships and sexual activity. Partners are often hesitant to resume sexual activity for fear of hurting the woman. There is concern that lovemaking may cause further injury or complications, such as pain or opening of the incision. Fear of contagion can also lead to impaired sexual interaction since physical contact may be avoided. It is interesting to note that in the late 19th century, oral-genital stimulation was thought to cause cancer.[9] In addition, because the surgical site is sensitive, partners often seek to protect the traumatized area.

Other partners are discomfited by their initial view of the incision, the flat or concave chest. The shock of this mutilation may be so startling that there is an aversive reaction. Scarring, particularly after radical mastectomy, can be frightening, and the sudden reality of a less than perfect body, traumatic. A partner's verbal acknowledgment of ambivalence toward the scar and willingness to explore these feelings with the woman can accelerate both parties' acceptance of the altered body image. If reticence and reluctance to initiate action by the partner continue without candid discussion, the woman may view such behavior as a confirmation of her undesirability and unworthiness as a love object.

One's sexual life prior to disability often determines sexual adjustment to chronic illness and the quality and frequency of activity after surgery.[10,11] If a woman did not previously realize her worth and value as a sexual being, then the assault to her self-image will probably be more severe after mastectomy. Women with little interest in sex prior to mastectomy use their surgery as a fortuitous event, excusing their participation in sexual activity.

The problems that a mastectomy presents may be magnified for the woman without a regular partner. Anticipation of sexual activity is often charged with intense anxiety, precipitating regression to the less threatening stage of adolescence. Activities such as hero worship of movie stars and athletes and the watching of soap operas may encourage vicarious sexual behavior through fantasy to the exclusion of sexual interaction. In the absence of a regular partner prior to mastectomy, a woman must deal with what and when to tell potential sexual partners. Frequently, relationships are terminated to avoid coping with growing intimacy and anticipated rejection. Other single women may seek repeated male validation of their desirability.

In addition to difficulties with a sexual partner, there may be strained relationships with children, particularly adolescent daughters. Since there is a genetic predisposition to breast cancer,[12,13] a mother may feel guilty about transmitting the "defective gene." Mastectomees with nubile adolescent daughters often find it difficult to deal with the contrast between their feelings of undesirability and their daughters' budding sexuality, the latter a constant reminder of potential loss of youth and attractiveness.

SUGGESTIONS FOR REMEDIATION OF PSYCHOSEXUAL PROBLEMS

Immediately following the body trauma of mastectomy and its attendant emotional problems, it is essential that open lines of communication be maintained between the woman, her sexual partner, family and professional helpers. Since many misconceptions arise from altered body image, candid discussion of these feelings can help minimize assaults on interpersonal relationships. Because of the mastectomee's fragile self-esteem, the postsurgical period is a time when she needs extra attention and love—when she can benefit from physical affection, tenderness and warmth from those who surround her.

Acknowledgment of the women as *a sexual being* by those who surround her in the hospital—professional helpers, sexual partner and family—can contribute to reducing anxiety. "Recognition by hospital staff that desire for sexual contact with one's partner is appropriate for the sick as well as the healthy may help relieve tension not only in patients but also in their spouses."[14]

Nurses can encourage patients to groom themselves and wear attractive lingerie rather than drab institutional garb. Since a woman is emotionally most vulnerable in the post-surgical period, physical contact can be an effective measure to counteract her threatened self-esteem.

Touching, tenderness and genuine warmth are especially important for sensory and emotional stimulation. Sexual partners can be physically affectionate, stroking their mates and making ribald remarks. A man who grins lecherously at his partner immediately after mastectomy may do more to bolster her morale than any therapeutic program.[15]

Hospital Care

Hospital-based social workers can engage in a variety of effective interventions to enhance a mastectomee's sexuality, including:

1. *Attendance to cosmetic needs*

a) A Reach to Recovery visit can be ordered through the local American Cancer Society unit. In this program, a medically stabilized mastectomy veteran visits women who have recently had a breast amputated. The visitor serves as an understanding, sensitive listener, sharing only that part of her experience that is pertinent to effecting the patient's recovery. The new mastectomee is presented with a dacron-filled temporary prosthesis that can be worn until her surgeon approves the purchase of a permanent one. Information is provided about the various types of prosthetic devices and bathing suits particularly suited to the mastectomee. In addition, patients are given a booklet dealing with the emotional issues of mastectomy as well as practical suggestions for post-surgical rehabilitation, e.g., illustrated exercises to restore physical functioning.

b) It is especially important that patients leave the hospital premises with at least a facade of femininity. If a Reach to Recovery visit is not possible, suggestions for fashioning a temporary prosthesis should be offered. A temporary prosthesis can be constructed from any soft material which, when inserted in a bra cup, will not provide any weight on the newly excised area, e.g., cotton filling from a sanitary napkin, wadded nylon hose or facial tissue.

2. *Provision for psychological support*

a) In addition to individual counseling, group counseling can be beneficial. Recognition that other women share the same confusion, distress and pain is especially supportive and may help decrease feelings of uniqueness and isolation. Themes for group discussions might include: feelings of bodily assault, fears of disease recurrence and premature death, problems of emotional adjustment to disfigurement and the impact of mastectomy on a woman's social network. The ther-

apeutic benefits of group support will hopefully include earlier confrontation and resolution of painful emotions as well
as increased communication with significant others.

b) If the sponsorship of such groups is not practical, the
availability of mastectomy consciousness-raising groups in
the community can be investigated.

Community Care

The most intense need for emotional support often emerges months
and sometimes years following discharge from the hospital. A mastectomee's rehabilitation can be facilitated through the support of community health agencies and professionals. Individual counseling,
relationship therapy, and group experience can be effective mechanisms
for obtaining information about breast cancer and its treatment as well
as working through painful feelings.

Community-based health professionals can teach the mastectomee a
range of exercises geared to developing a sense of heightened body awareness and to restoring confidence as a sexual being. A variety of individual
and group techniques can be suggested, but a combination will be most
effective. Some of these exercises are best done in the nude.

Exercises to be done in private include the following:

1. *Water Play* — Water play can be used to increase sensory
   discrimination, stimulate sexual arousal and release sexual
   tension. Lying in a warm bubble bath or standing in a shower,
   gently soaping the entire body surface, is a non-threatening
   means of tactile exploration of one's own body and can be
   less intimidating to those women unaccustomed to self-pleasuring. Altering water pressure with a shower massage to sore
   or tense areas may be both pleasurable and soothing. Practicing repeated contraction and relaxation of different muscles
   (thigh, pelvis, abdomen or buttocks) can be sexually arousing
   for some women.

2. *Mirror-Image*

   a) By posing before a mirror in various gradients of light,
   ranging from dim to bright sunlight and regulating the amount
   of light to the optimal level of comfort, a woman can progressively desensitize her reactions and explore feelings about her
   altered body image.

   b) Standing before a full-length mirror, preferably a three-
   paneled one, the woman articulates her feelings about the aes-
   thetics and function of each body part. By this means, she can
   increase her self-awareness of positive as well as negative

feelings. With each subsequent exposure, disparity between her expectations and reality is reduced.

3. *Role-Playing* — By repetitively role-playing her concept of the ideal feminine image, a woman may gradually incorporate some of the admired traits as part of her new self-concept.

4. *Personification* (Gestalt technique) — By holding a two-way conversation with her missing breast, reviewing the significant role her breasts played in her life, e.g., wearing her first bra, initial experiences in sex play and breast feeding, the mourning process can be facilitated.

Group exercises include the following:

1. *Body-Meditation* — Lying in a comfortable position, fully clothed and with eyes closed, women are instructed to touch, massage and caress those parts of their bodies that conjure up negative feelings. After completion of the exercise, the support provided by group feedback will contribute to the dissipation of such feelings.

2. *Human-Figure Drawing* — Women are given a lapboard, colored markers and paper. Each is instructed to draw her own image. The drawings are then passed to other group members, each of whom writes her interpretation of the feelings expressed by the figure in the picture. The drawing is returned to its creator, who then talks about what she intended to express and her reactions to the group's comments. This exercise is particularly effective for those women who are unwilling or unable to articulate their feelings.

3. *Mirror-Image* — The body image exercise done in private before a three-way mirror is equally effective when executed individually in front of a group. This exercise provides many women with their first socially nude experience and is a prime opportunity for viewing other mastectomees. Looking at others with their explicit permission in a safe, structured setting is beneficial for gaining a perspective of one's body contours in relation to others. Because the affected site is always hidden from others' view, women imagine that their own mutilation is unique and much worse than that of others who have had the same surgery.

Reorientation to Self

It is especially important, if there are children in the household, that the woman and her partner have the opportunity to spend time alone after the mastectomy. Since the mastectomee is often surrounded by friends and relatives upon hospital discharge, periods of privacy are essential for the couple's psychological adjustment to the situation. Time is needed for them to discuss their feelings, expectations, as well as this new body.

Some women are distressed at finding themselves appearing nippleless when wearing a prosthesis. This can be a disconcerting problem particularly in regard to today's fashion of wearing soft bras, which give the illusion of being braless. Simple and inexpensive devices, such as "pasties," buttons or balled fringe trimming, can be inserted in the bra to correct for this deficit,[16] and thus enhance the woman's sense of femininity.

When the postoperative site is stimulated, many women experience a strange tactile sensation owing to varying degrees of numbness in the area. If viewed positively rather than fearfully, this unfamiliar feeling can be recognized as creating a new erogenous zone. As a woman becomes more comfortable with herself as a viable sexual being, she will begin to appreciate this new sensual pleasure. Refraining temporarily from coitus can be encouraged to permit concentration on touching and cuddling. The numbness will gradually recede and new erotic arousal will result in feelings of warmth, affection and closeness between the partners.

Other problems that seemingly interfere with resuming sexual relations can be resolved if given careful thought. For example, women who are fearful that sexual performance will aggravate their surgical wound can use a pillow as a protective device. Some mastectomees are more comfortable wearing a prosthesis and bra during lovemaking. Also, in the case of metastatic disease, specifically a lesion in the pubic bone, awareness of pain can be reduced if coitus is executed in other than the missionary position, e.g., rear entry, scissors or female superior.

In instances where a woman's revulsion to her surgical site is so intense that it impedes her performing monthly self-examinations of the chest wall, one effective technique may be to enlist participation of her sex partner. Natural concomitants of his gentle assay would be pleasurable, sensual and possibly erotic. At the same time, the partner communicates to the woman that she is accepted, which in turn might hasten the return of a strong sense of self-esteem and joyous intimacy. The sharing of a task often relieves the ambivalence between one's taking total responsibility for health and the desire to force others to assume this burden.

Healthy adjustment to chronic illness is a process that demands the energies and talent of all community resources if quality care is desired. Therefore, it is essential that long-term services be available.

SEXUAL PROBLEMS FROM THE HEALTH PRACTITIONER'S PERSPECTIVE

Despite the growing openness about sexuality, health care workers have not done enough to help mastectomees. Generally, such personnel are ill-prepared and uncomfortable talking about sex and hence, do not routinely encourage discussion. Professionals suffer from what Gochros has called "sexual blinders."[17] Various rationalizations are used to mask resistance and inadequacy in dealing with sexual problems. Consequently, women who are quick to detect this discomfort will be reluctant to pursue the subject.

NEED FOR SEX EDUCATION

Although responsibility for sexual problems has traditionally been relegated to the medical sphere, health personnel, including physicians, generally are unable to treat their mastectomy patients' sexual problems because of inadequate preparation in their professional training.[18] Incomplete knowledge about human sexual responses and personal awkwardness and discomfort have caused sexual issues to be devalued or avoided. Approaching sexual matters with patients can be threatening when vulnerability to their personal experiences is awakened.[19] At the same time, some patients are reluctant to confide for fear of adverse judgment or condemnation. Consequently, a conspiracy of silence is often maintained.

Greater awareness of iatrogenic sexual dysfunction is needed. Before professionals can realistically be expected to assist women with the emotional turmoil induced by mastectomy, skill, competence and sophistication in human sexuality are required. In addition, while facilitating an atmosphere of permissiveness, professionals who convey comfort with their own sexuality can serve as role models for patients and help put them at ease. The content for any human sexuality curriculum should include treating sexual dysfunction in the acutely and chronically ill, the unabled and disfigured as well as in the able-bodied. Emphasis on prevention of sexual dysfunction is also appropriate. Various techniques can be used to accomplish these tasks, including small-group discussion, role-playing, desensitization-resensitization and audiovisual presentations (explicit movies made specifically for teaching situations).[20] These films illustrate the male and female sexual responses, sensate focus exercises, coital positions, self-pleasuring, homosexual relationships and sexual mythologies. The result of this process is a new and heightened awareness of one's own sexuality and appreciation of the meaning and significance of a joyous and loving relationship.[21] Unless professionals are provided with an adequate education in sexuality, they will continue to be inattentive to patients' sexual problems, and thus perpetuate the pervasive inadequacy that is characteristic of the medical model.

WHAT CAN SOCIAL WORKERS DO?

Since responsibility for patients' sexual well-being is not yet being fully assumed by the medical profession, social workers can make a unique contribution to patient care by considering this as being within their legitimate domain. With their skills and training in psychosocial diagnosis and assessment, social workers are particularly well-equipped to play an instrumental role in sexual counseling. Although some social workers are already engaged in this activity, we advocate its inclusion as integral to social work practice in the health care field. Social workers must first evaluate the existence of sexual problems by introducing the subject with the woman and her partner, each separately, followed by conjoint interviews. At the same time, the patient and her partner must develop confidence and trust in the social worker before their inhibitions can be overcome. Yet even when tact is employed, some clients will censor their responses.

Topics to be covered include:
1. Daily living patterns
2. Involvement in social activities
3. Availability of social support systems
4. Emotional status
5. Degree of physical intimacy exclusive of lovemaking
6. Possible discrepancies between performance and expectation
7. Frequency of intercourse and other forms of lovemaking
8. Modalities of expression in their sexual repertoire
9. The nature of the marital or other intimate relationships

Assessment of self-concept and body image is vital. Since the woman's sex partner is involved in her impaired sexuality and responds to her feelings of inadequacy, it is important that he be included in any plan for counseling. An hour of candid discussion when the diagnosis is established may be far more advantageous to the patient and her partner than three months of psychotherapy during and after treatment.[7] Providing a non-judgmental atmosphere will encourage greater candor. Nonthreatening self-disclosure provides a comfortable, safe environment in which a client can begin to deal more effectively with her problems. In addition, assurances of confidentiality may decrease nonresponse rates to sensitive items such as sexual behavior.[22]

Knowledge about human sexual responses and dysfunctions, as well as the psychologic and social components of sexuality, is essential to prepare workers to be comfortable with their own sexuality. Such ease will enable them to elicit information more readily, and to counsel from the client's perspective rather than from that of the dominant cultural value system. Training in human sexuality, preferably with experiential exercises, is essential for medical social work staff development programs. Ideally, sexuality training should be initiated prior to in-service education, and considered as an integral component of social work curricula. This will equip social workers to be increasingly aware of their own sexual attitudes and practices and therefore more sensitive to the needs of their clients. Another aim of this sexual education process is developing skill and competence in conversing frankly about sex. As Salhoot states: "In a counseling situation, we are not only therapist to client, but one sexual human being to another sexual human being."[21]

RESEARCH PERSPECTIVES

Although the literature has traditionally treated sexual dysfunction with a psychoanalytic interpretation, there has been a recent shift toward emphasizing the value of the quality of human interactions.[23] Objective measures of sexuality are most often limited to frequency of coitus and orgasm, number of sexual partners,[24] or by the couple's expressed satisfaction with the sexual relationship. Many studies fallaciously assume that the woman has access to a suitable partner. As Griffith and Trieschmann suggest, we must be careful to divorce desire from opportunity.[25] At the same time, we must realize that copulation is not the only way to express love and affection. Traditional indices of sexuality and sexual dysfunction must be expanded to include evaluation of self-concept, body-image and affective bonds of marital and other intimate relationships. At the same time, since different meanings have been applied to the term *self-concept*, standardized definitions are essential for reducing non-equivalency of measures. Without conceptual clarity, operationalizing constructs becomes an impossible task for the researcher.[26] The excessive focus on performance as a standard of sexual adjustment needs to be replaced by greater emphasis on other modalities of sexual expression in interpersonal relationships; thus a sharp distinction between expressions of sensuality and copulation would be made. Evaluating behavioral patterns of mastectomees and their sexual partners both independently and together provides a simple way to cross-validate couples' reports, and therefore check for consistency of responses.

If the goal of the research study is to identify problems which disturb a couple's relationship, sex history questionnaires should probe sexual functioning within an interactional context rather than focus on psychological states and historical performance. Lacking objective standards of "normal" sexual behavior, dysfunction can be assessed only in relation to congruency between a couple's actual and expected relationship.[27] A sex questionnaire should include items exploring desire for and frequency of extramarital affairs, obsession with breasts, attitudes of both sex partners toward their relationship and their concomitant physical expression, factors which inhibit or impede communication, reactions to rejection, attitudes and values about sex, and the frequency, manifestation and duration of male sexual dysfunction resulting from his partner's mastectomy. Triangulation of methods, such as a combination of interview-questionnaires and observations of subject interactions during mastectomy consciousness-raising or marital-counseling group sessions, has the added features of obtaining data that are not otherwise elicited, thus enabling more accurate recording of information.

Finally, whatever method is chosen, the investigator involved in sensitive topics of research is confronted with an ethical issue. Since questions can potentially increase a respondent's awareness of problems, and therefore raise levels of anxiety, some participants may request therapeutic assistance from the interviewer. Although the research team may be tempted to provide the help, such action could seriously bias the study's outcome. This is not to imply, however, that support should be denied in an obvious situation of crisis. Since the deliberate probing of sensitive psychological areas might open Pandora's box, there is a moral obligation that some mechanism for counseling distraught subjects be provided. One alternative might be to hire a social worker to either offer direct service or to make referrals to appropriate mental health professionals, agencies or self-help organizations.

It is important that social workers recognize that research is a legitimate area of social work practice. Although patient responsibilities often make it difficult for clinicians to realize the potential contribution of research to their professional practice, it is time to set priorities. Benign neglect and apathy should no longer be tolerated. Research of the sexual concerns of the chronically ill is especially important. Since candid discussions about sex have become more culturally acceptable, social workers and other health professionals are called upon more frequently to counsel patients on this subject. In the final analysis, research can be valuable in determining additional patient vulnerabilities requiring professional psychologic assistance, modes of therapeutic intervention, expanded roles for social workers in treating sexual dysfunction, and the effectiveness of sex training programs on professional counseling. It should also increase our understanding of the effects of a mastectomy on a woman, her sexual partner and their interrelationship.

CONCLUSION

Ideally, treatment of sexual dysfunction after mastectomy should be a team approach. All caregivers should be able to respond to the patient's pressing anxieties when they arise.[28] The social worker can serve as an intermediary between the woman and her physician. Among other responsibilities, he or she can assist the patient to cope with any sexual inadequacy by giving the couple an opportunity to express discomfort. When appropriate, referrals should be made to professionals with sex counseling expertise.

Regarding self-image, cancer must be seen as a state of being specifically affecting the physical state of health, rather than as an indelible imprint on one's character or inner sense of psychological well-being. The loss of a breast does not change a woman's value as a person. If not properly dealt with, such mutilation may interfere with self-esteem, impair interpersonal relationships and precipitate sexual dissatisfaction.

Social workers can make a significant contribution to post-mastectomy rehabilitation by offering services designed to facilitate women's acceptance of their altered body image and worth as sexual beings. In particular, it is desirable that programs aim to increase sexual enjoyment, reduce the focus on performance expectations, explore non-coital techniques and enhance communication with partners. At the same time, professionals should not be overzealous in attributing sexual concerns to mastectomees since some women can effectively cope on their own.[29]

With increased orientation toward holistic patient care, circumvention or avoidance of the sexual needs of mastectomees can no longer be justified. If health care professionals are to ease their burden, they have little recourse but to accept the responsibility for sex counseling as a legitimate professional endeavor.

REFERENCES

1. Wasow, M. Human sexuality and terminal illness. Health Social Work 2:105, 1977.
2. Mann, J. Is sex counseling here to stay? Counseling Psychologist 5:60, 1975.
3. Gagnon, J. H. and Simon, W. S. Sexual Conduct: The Social Sources of Human Sexuality. Chicago, Aldine Publ. Co., 1973.
4. Barker, R. G. Adjustment to Physical Handicap and Illness: A Survey of the Social Psychology of Physique and Disability. New York, Social Science Res. Council, 1953.
5. Tyler, E. A. Disfigurement and sexual behavior. Med. Aspects Hum. Sexuality 9:77, 1975.
6. Ford, A. B. and Orfirer, A. P. Sexual behavior and the chronically ill patient. Med. Aspects Hum. Sexuality 1:51, 1967.

7. Bard, M. and Sutherland, A. Adaptation to Radical Mastectomy. *In* The Psychological Impact of Cancer, American Cancer Society (Ed.), 1974, pp. 55-71.

8. Kaplan, H. S. The New Sex Therapy. New York, Brunner/Mazel in cooperation with Quadrangle/The New York Times Book Co., 1974.

9. Bergeret, L. F. E. The Preventive Obstacle or Conjugal Onanism. New York, Turner and Mignard, 1898.

10. Sutherland, A. M. and Orbach, C. E. Psychological impact of cancer and cancer surgery. II. Depressive reactions associated with surgery for cancer. Cancer 5:857, 1952.

11. Schoenberg, B. and Carr, A. C. Loss of External Organs: Limb Amputation, Mastectomy, and Disfiguration. *In* Loss and Grief: Psychological Management in Medical Practice (Schoenberg et al., Eds.) New York, Columbia Univ. Press, 1970, pp. 119-131.

12. Papaioannou, A. N. The Etiology of Human Breast Cancer. New York, Springer-Verlag, 1974.

13. Anderson, D. E. Familial and Genetic Predisposition. *In* Risk Factors in Breast Cancer (B. A. Stoll, Ed.) London, William Heinemann Medical Books Ltd., 1976, pp. 3-24.

14. Leiber, L., Plumb, M. M., Gerstenzang, M. L. and Holland, J. The communication of affection between cancer patients and their spouses. Psychosomat. Med. 38:387, 1976.

15. Klagsbrun, S. Communications in the treatment of cancer. Am. J. Nursing 71:944, 1971.

16. Rollin, B. First, You Cry. Philadelphia, J. B. Lippincott, 1976.

17. Gochros, H. L. Social Work's Sexual Blinders. *In* Human Sexuality and Social Work (Gochros and Schultz, Eds.) New York, Association Press, 1972, pp. 85-91.

18. Pauly, I. B. and Goldstein, S. G. Physicians' ability to treat sexual problems. Med. Aspects Hum. Sexuality 4:24;30-33;38;40;45-46;49, 1970.

19. Golden, J. S. Management of sexual problems by the physician. Obstet. Gynec. 23:471, 1964.

20. Lief, H. I. and Karlen, A. (Eds.) Sex Education in Medicine. New York, Spectrum Publications, 1976.

21. Salhoot, J. T. Human Caring and Sexuality in Chronic Illness. Paper presented at the 14th Annual Institute for Social Workers, Los Angeles, Calif., 1974.

22. Singer, E. Informed consent: consequences for response rate and response quality in social surveys. Am. Sociol. Rev. 43:144, 1978.

23. Kirkendall, L. A. and Libby, R. W. Interpersonal Relationships—Crux of the Sexual Renaissance. *In* Sexual Development and Behavior: Selected Readings (A. M. Juhasz, Ed.) Homewood, Ill., The Dorsey Press, 1973, pp. 264-278.

24. Dlin, B. M., Perlman, A. and Ringold, E. Psychosexual response to ileostomy and colostomy. Am. J. Psychiat. 126:374, 1969.

25. Griffith, E. R. and Trieschmann, R. B. Sexual functioning in women with spinal cord injury. Arch. Phys. Med. Rehab. 56:18, 1975.

26. Wells, L. E. and Marwell, G. Self-Esteem: Its Conceptualization and Measurement. Beverly Hills, Calif., Sage Publications, 1976.
27. Lo Piccolo, J. and Steger, J. C. The sexual interaction inventory: A new instrument for assessment of sexual dysfunction. Arch. Sexual Behav. 3:585, 1974.
28. Jaffe, L. The Terminally Ill. *In* The Sexually Oppressed (Gochros and Gochros, Eds.) New York, Association Press, 1977, pp. 277-292.
29. Diamond, M. Sexuality and the Handicapped. *In* Social and Psychological Aspects of Disability (J. Stubbins, Ed.) Baltimore, University Park Press, 1977, pp. 439-450.

17

Counseling in Mastectomy

ALEX COMFORT, M.B.

So long as breast cancer remains common in healthy women, and radical mastectomy remains a common treatment, any woman may be confronted by its psychic effects on body image, self-esteem, and sexual self-image. The prevention of these is an important part of rehabilitation.

Women patients who have no breast problem should be encouraged to discuss breast cancer with their regular physician. It may never occur, but if it does, prior discussion of the facts on treatment, the options available, and the physician's probable advice, will avoid the need to make decisions in a panic situation. Such a dialogue is essential to informed consent—which is in fact lacking in many cases of radical mastectomy. During a prior discussion, the arguments for and against radical surgery, conservative surgery ("lumpectomy"), radiotherapy, and plastic reconstruction can be reviewed, so that any contingency can be faced from prepared positions. A leaflet proposing such a discussion in non-threatening terms can be made available in the office or billing department.

MODEL LEAFLET

Breast cancer is by no means rare, and you have been advised of the desirability of self-examination to detect its early signs.

Another precaution, less usually recommended but which we feel to be very worthwhile, is that you make an appointment with a member of this practice to talk about breast cancer and its treatment.

Though there is no reason to believe that you will ever have breast cancer, it is a sensible precaution, like having an insurance policy, to talk over with your doctor the options that exist in treating this disease while you are perfectly well. The reason for this is that if the problem ever arose, you would know what means are available to deal with it, as well as the general principles on which you would be advised by your surgeon, rather than having to consider them under the stress of urgency and emergency.

Although some people feel a little superstitious about discussing an unpleasant contingency which will probably never happen, insurance does not cause accidents. As your physicians, we like to be sure that if we were ever in the position of having to advise you in a matter which might involve radical surgery, you would fully understand all the alternatives, and the reasons why we urge one of them rather than another. If we have had the opportunity of such a discussion with you when there is no immediate problem, it will avoid the need for sudden choices if the problem were to arise. Moreover, many women find that far from causing worry, a sensible precautionary discussion of this kind, in which they can express their feelings and wishes to their physician, is in fact reassuring—simply because it is reassuring to know that if an emergency arises, you have had ample time to develop with us a strategy for dealing with it and will not be "railroaded" into surgery.

If you wish to act on this idea, please tell the receptionist that you would like an appointment for this purpose, so that adequate time can be set aside.

When the contingency arises, a psychotherapeutic dimension is invariably opened. However urgent the surgery, it is mandatory that the patient have the opportunity of facing, with skilled help, her fears, her anger and her changed self-image.

In women who have a male partner, this therapy must extend to both individuals who should be seen both separately and together. The woman will feel herself to be mutilated. She may fear sexual rejection even when it is not present, and interpret any denial by her partner as a cover-up. Men may be profoundly disturbed by the altered image as much as by the fact of the anatomic changes involved. They may in effect be irrationally rejecting, or denying rejection, or simply projecting their own embarrassment. No surgery which leaves this situation without skilled help can be regarded as completed surgery.

The psychotherapist should assess the best means of enabling these feelings to be faced. In most cases photographs of the longterm post-operative result, clothed and unclothed, help to reduce the anxiety of both partners to realistic levels; in other cases, it helps if the husband is encouraged to assist with the dressings. As in all cases of extensive sur-gery, it is of value to have available volunteers who have themselves undergone surgery and have adjusted. Wherever possible, a group ther-apy program should be maintained in which immediately post-operative, convalescent and recovered patients and couples take part, since those who have dealt with the problem are valuable sources of practical advice as well as reducers of anxiety by example.

Psychosexual sequelae can be minimized by 1) early counseling and 2) practical advice. For example, if the couple's sleeping position has made the excised breast also the one most accessible for an approach to lovemaking, they may be advised to change sides: however, the fact of sleeping on the unaccustomed side of a partner can interfere with some men's sexual performance if it is strongly patterned on habit, and the failure is then interpreted by both partners as rejection.

Single women who have had a mastectomy sometimes withdraw al-together from sexual contacts, or compensate by becoming promiscu-ous beyond their normal pattern of acceptance in the pursuit of reassurance. A good counseling tactic in discussing future sexual activi-ties is to warn against these overreactions and to develop a strategy for the dating situation. The patient who dates a man and feels the situ-ation to be one in which—preoperatively—she would have welcomed lovemaking, should tell the man conversationally that she has had a mastectomy, and treat any nonrenewal or nonpursuit of advances exactly as she would have preoperatively, as simply failure to follow through. Insofar as it relates to her surgery, it suggests that the man may have been too unsure of himself to accept the situation, or more often, too unsure of how to handle it without embarrassment to her—a basi-cally caring, rather than a rejecting, response. She must attempt to ac-quire the skill of conveying that she is not embarrassed and does not invite rejection or consider herself sexually disqualified, which she is not. It is important that she tell the man on *which side* the surgery was performed, and repeat the information. If the relationship proceeds, she may volunteer that he "be extra kind to the other one." If intercourse seems likely, she should specifically say: "I can keep my bra on if you like, or not" or go along with any suggestion that they commence inter-course in the dark.

The importance for her orientation is that she recognizes that she is not overcoming any drawback in herself, but acting as therapist to her part-ner's fear of saying the wrong thing, and in doing this she should offer leads for him to follow. She should discuss with the counselor any fears concerning what may happen, any anxiety over the likelihood of "charity humps," and the host of other fears which go with the loss of a socially overrated sexual asset. Insight into likely male reactions, and the fact that these reactions are far more likely to be concerned and reticent than rejecting, can help a great deal—most of all if the therapist herself has had a mastectomy and can speak from experience. Only after all these fears have been faced, and couple communication has been fully tested in married patients and sexual willingness in single, should it be pointed out that the sensitivity originally present in the intact breast is very often transferred to the mastectomy scar; it may even be heightened, so that light touching with the fingertips while the intact breast, skin and clitoris are stimulated can produce extremely intense arousal.

Every radical breast surgery which fails to include a full program of personal and sexual rehabilitation can be counted inadequate. The counselor may be the family physician if experientially qualified, a psychotherapist, or a professionally led volunteer program; but the counselor should be prepared to handle not only normal disturbance over a traumatic event, but also acute depression, carcinophobia, and the added sequelae of radical treatments such as chemotherapy involving loss of hair or radiotherapy which may affect libido. The responsible surgeon cannot unload responsibility on an unsupervised group. In some cases he may find it helpful to discuss his own attitudes toward surgery which affects the sexual image of woman with a psychiatric colleague, a procedure which might reduce the statistically unjustified frequency of radical surgery and increase the acceptance of conservative methods and reconstructive operations.

18

Miscellaneous Medical and Surgical Conditions

ALEX COMFORT, M.B.

Any condition which impairs the specific "athletic" requirements of intercourse can produce sexual dysfunction. Aside from pain and motor disorder, the aspect of sexual function which most commonly causes problems is the overbreathing which accompanies the final stages of arousal and climax. Any problem which produces dyspnea will surface at this time. Inquiry into "loss of sexual interest" will quite often reveal that either the subject becomes breathless, or that climax is prevented by uncontrollable coughing. In particular, *exercise-induced asthma* can be sexually disabling. Symington and Kerr[3] found that while this common problem in both sexes could be elicited on inquiry, it was rarely volunteered. Hyperventilation, anxiety, and possibly the stirring-up of bed-dust containing house-mite débris and other allergens can all contribute to the symptom; it responds well to prophylactic treatment and should be specifically inquired about in asthmatics.

The tachycardia and increased blood pressure of orgasm do not as a rule give rise to dysfunction, except in patients already anxious about cardiac function, for whom these effects can be totally disabling. Heart attack and stroke are not common during intercourse (they more commonly occur during detumescence). Persistent headache beginning during intercourse should be investigated. The brief "loading" of the heart involved in normal intercourse is probably too brief, unless orgasm is frequent, to act as a prophylactic against heart disease, but its effects are more likely to be beneficial than harmful. Where arrhythmias (especially paroxysmal tachycardia) originate during intercourse, they appear to correlate more with anxiety than with exertion.

One group of problems may arise from the difficulty of discriminating between the manifestations of orgasm and those of illness. Normal people may exhibit trismus, convulsions, or apparent loss of consciousness as a regular feature of sexual climax, and the muscular contractions can be sufficiently violent to give rise to stiffness. It is difficult to discriminate this highly motor reaction from instances in which orgasm merges with epilepsy: the best discriminants are 1) the history—patients are aware of their own response pattern, and 2) the relatively rapid recovery in view of the apparent severity of the discharge.

Urination at climax is not rare in women, with or without loss of consciousness; in others, apparent collapse can alarm a partner who is unaccustomed to it. Neither of these is an indication of pathology, but if confusion persists after recovery, something more than orgasm has occurred. Grand mal and temporal lobe epilepsy, as well as rarer attacks (narcolepsy, catalepsy) can coincide with orgasm, either regularly or on occasion. It is important to note that in spite of its spectacular character, orgasm is a particularly safe form of exertion—statistics indicate that guilt or anxiety are more hazardous stresses than sexual climax.

In dealing with major neurological diseases, impairment of erection depends on impairment of sensory and autonomic paths almost exclusively; thus rigidity may impair sexual function in parkinsonism, but erection is usually unaffected except in the rarer, autonomic-centered form (Shy-Drager syndrome). Impotence is absent in amyotrophic lateral sclerosis, paralleling the absence of bedsores in this condition. In one case of terminal paralysis from this cause, erection and ejaculation persisted until at least three months before death.[2]

The impotence of diabetics may involve vascular, neuroendocrine or neural elements, but substantial functional elements (anxiety, alcohol, anger) very often contribute to it. Trial of bromocriptine, on the assumption that impotency may parallel hyperprolactinemia, both in diabetes and in the sexual dysfunction accompanying dialysis, has produced disappointing results.

SURGICAL CONDITIONS

The combination of physical interference, loss of confidence and "desexing" by a mutilating or unesthetic procedure is common to all extensive surgery. The following example of ileostomy illustrates the factors involved.

In a survey of 303 married ileostomy patients, Burnham et al.[1] found that ileostomy without rectal excision caused no sexual dysfunction in either sex, and that only 8 per cent encountered practical difficulties in intercourse. Some 30 per cent experienced "embarrassment" about their condition; 10 per cent attributed some marital tension, and 2 per cent marital breakdown, to the stoma. Rectal excision produced impotence or other sexual dysfunction in 29 per cent of men—among those up to 35 years old, 5 experienced partial and none total erectile incompetence, but 9 out of 61 had ejaculatory impotence. In the group aged 36-45, 11 out of 30 had partial and 5 had total erectile incompetence, but function continued to improve two years after operation. Orgasm in women was unaffected by rectal excision, but 30 per cent reported dyspareunia.

In all such procedures, regardless of severity, preoperative attitude, preoperative education where possible, careful assessment of the physiological deficit by measurement, individual postoperative psychotherapy of both patient and partner, and the use of group support, contribute to the outcome. Therapy groups should exist in all major surgical centers for follow-up and adjustment, and sexual problems should be included in their agenda. Such groups will contain recently operated, convalescent and long postoperative patients under the direction of a skilled moderator. Their potential for mutual support in all areas of postoperative living is immense. No patient subjected to mutilating surgery should be discharged home without strong encouragement to join such a group; participation can be prepared immediately after operation by the use of tapes or bedside visits.

THE AMPUTEE

The amputee acquires disability late (often very late) in life, and the sense of castration or mutilation is therefore a predominant problem in both sexes. Much of what has been written about mastectomy applies with equal force to limb amputation, in regard to self-image, partner reaction, and access to support and reassurance from persons who have undergone similar surgery. There are also practical problems which may interfere with sexuality by upsetting established patterns of coital behavior; interference with balance (in leg amputees) and the existence of a painful phantom, or of pain in the phantom at orgasm, are reasonably common complaints.

Rehabilitation programs have been short on the sexual aspects of the rehabilitative process, partly because of the high age of many amputees for nontraumatic pathologies and the mythology of asexual aging. The essentials are to establish the preoperative level of sexual function, to give opportunity and encouragement for sexual as well as occupational and other anxieties to be ventilated, to organize early discussion with other patients—preferably other couples—who have had similar surgery, and to inquire into sexual function during the process of rehabilitation. The woman with a good prosthesis is in much the same psychological situation as that described for the mastectomy patient; concealed disability may produce more serious psychosexual difficulties than overt, because it has at some time during intimacy to be unveiled. The amputated male, aside from "castration anxiety" is commonly, and realistically, less preoccupied that sexual competency will be impaired (the "wounded soldier ploy," as one patient accurately described it). If women respond positively to the "wounded soldier" (who may himself not appreciate or admit the fact), women amputees need to be aware that amputation itself is a powerful psychosexual mode of release for some males, ranging in intensity from a preference to a completely preoccupying fetish. The desirability of sexual attraction based on such a preference would need to be assessed in the particular case; since all human psychosexual preferences appear to arise at a pre-rational level, there is no prima facie reason to reject it, but premarital discussion by both parties with an experienced counselor would appear to be wise.

Problems arising from high lower-limb amputations in either sex may involve experimenting with coital posture, e.g., loss of an upper limb may require change of sleeping-side. Loss of both upper limbs carries the serious disability of interfering with masturbation, especially in males, not all of whom can "convert" from manual to pillow friction. The problem should be specifically addressed—prostheses are not made with this application in mind. Some patients have found that foam-rubber sleeves fitted to both jaws of a split-hook prosthesis are effective for this purpose.

As with all other sexual disabilities, the mechanical problems of loss of limb are superable by ingenuity and improvisation. It is the psychosocial pressures—the equivalents of sorcery in primitive orders—which are the main source of functional disability, and it is these that the preoperative, postoperative and rehabilitation staffs must join forces to detect and exorcise.

TERMINAL ILLNESS

The phases of coming to terms with death include denial, anger, depression and acceptance. Individual response will differ, apart from the specific effects of illness and medication. Some patients may respond by total sexual withdrawal, others by acting-out and hypersexuality. The phase of acceptance often includes a drawing-together of spouses in a particularly deep sexual communion. In some cases elaborate deception may be taking place. A wife may induce her husband to seek sex counseling because of impotence, and the husband may then inform the therapist that he is concealing a diagnosis of malignancy or leukemia from his family. Exactly as in catastrophic surgery, and with even deeper psychological consequences, group support by way of a therapy group is of immense value to the dying patient and to those around him or her. When death itself must be addressed, whether at home or in the hospital, the physician should ensure the opportunity for continued sexual intimacy as a natural part of leavetaking, a sensitivity which hospitals sometimes omit to honor.

REFERENCES

1. Burnham, W.D., Lennard-Brown, J.E. and Brooke, B.N. Gut 17:391, 1976.
2. Jokelainen, M. and Palo, J. Lancet 1:1246, 1976.
3. Symington, I. and Kerr, J.W. Lancet 2:693, 1976.

19

Sex Prosthetics

WILLIAM L. FURLOW, M.D., F.A.C.S.

Physicians have long searched for a suitable method of surgical treatment of the impotent male, recognizing that there are numerous causes of impotence, not all of which are amenable to psychiatric counseling and sex therapy. For a sizeable group of patients it was necessary to devise a surgical means whereby the flaccid penis could be made erect and therefore suitable for vaginal penetration during sexual intercourse. To this end, a suitable prosthetic device must be easy to implant, acceptable to tissue, and tolerable to the patient. This chapter will endeavor to cover the subject of sex prosthetic devices currently in use for the surgical correction of male impotence, including indications, guidelines for evaluation and selection of patients, and evaluation of the implantable devices presently used to restore sexual function.

DEFINITION OF IMPOTENCE

The patient who complains of impotence is generally considered unable to develop an erection suitable for vaginal penetration and the act of sexual intercourse. This is only one form of impotence, however. It is only through careful questioning that the physician learns about those patients who consider themselves impotent because they are unable to maintain a suitable erection as a result of premature ejaculation, and therefore find themselves unable to continue intercourse for the purpose of bringing their partner to a climax. This type of patient rarely requires initial surgical treatment, and he certainly should be encouraged to seek sexual counseling from a qualified sex therapist. Occasionally, some of these patients will be refractory to psychiatric treatment and they are then referred to the urologist as a candidate for implantation of a penile prosthesis.

Another group of patients often seen by us are men who state that they can develop a partial erection that may be suitable for vaginal penetration only with the use of manual methods to maintain vaginal contact. These practices are generally undesirable to both the patient and his partner and hence these persons seek consultation in search of a method whereby the penis can be made erect and rigid. The cause may be either organic or psychogenic.

INDICATIONS FOR PENILE IMPLANTATION

The patient who seeks surgical help to correct his impotence is generally a highly motivated person who has strong inner stimulation to make himself whole once more. Such a patient may be impotent for a variety of reasons. Table 1 outlines the causative factors associated with impotence. It should be noted that I have divided impotence into three general categories: psychogenic, physiologic, and organic.

Table 1. Causes of Male Impotence

I. Organic impotence
    Diabetes mellitus
    Diabetic neuropathy
    Alcoholism
    Drug abuse
    Drug side effects (guanethidine, spironolactone, anticholinergics,
       reserpine, estrogen, methadone)
    Vascular diseases (aorta and iliac arteries)
    Endocrinologic disorders (acromegaly)
    Addison's disease
    Adrenal neoplasia
    Hypogonadism
    Myxedema
    Hyperthyroidism
    Neurologic diseases (multiple sclerosis, amyotrophic lateral sclerosis,
       temporal lobe lesions, pernicious anemia, nutritional deficiencies)
    Urologic problems (Peyronie's disease, hydrocele, varicocele, priapism)
    Complication of surgical procedures
    Trauma

II. Psychogenic impotence

III. Physiologic impotence

In my opinion, certain patients may be impotent only as a result of the natural aging process. I speak specifically about the healthy male between the ages of 60 and 75 years who has neither organic nor psychogenic impotence but is nonetheless unable to develop an erection despite strong motivation and desire. Such a patient might best be classified as physiologically impotent.

GUIDELINES FOR PATIENT EVALUATION AND SELECTION

I believe that we as physicians concerned with the treatment of impotence owe much to the lay publications, which were among the first to deal with the subject of impotence in an open and frank fashion. Sensitive articles on this subject have played an important role in educating the public. In addition, this circumstance has caused many physicians to revise their own approach to the discussions of impotence with their patients. By conservative estimate, 50 per cent of the patients with this problem seen by me at the Mayo Clinic are self-referred, having acquired initial knowledge of the surgical techniques employed through newspaper and magazine articles.

The result has been a definite need to establish specific guidelines for patient selection for surgical implantation. Those guidelines are outlined in Table 2.

Table 2. The Inflatable Penile Prosthesis: Essentials in Patient Selection

---

Historical aspects of impotence
Total vs. partial impotence
Discussion of device; function; demonstration
(with patient and spouse or partner)
Female partner acceptance
MMPI evaluation
Psychologic evaluation
Motivation
NPT Monitor

Causative Factors. The historical events leading to the onset of the patient's impotence should be established so that his sexual dysfunction can be classified. As mentioned, it is helpful to place a particular case of impotence into the psychogenic, physiologic, or organic category; this may not always be possible, but one should try. This portion of the evaluation should include all treatment methods previously employed to correct the patient's impotence and the results of such treatment. From this information the physician will discover some very necessary and useful information as to the patient's motivation and that of his wife which will help him to decide whether the patient is a suitable candidate for penile implantation. In my opinion, it is essential that the married man's wife be in full agreement with the patient's desires to undergo surgical treatment.

It is also assumed that the physician will have carefully evaluated the status of those organic problems thought to be the cause of the patient's sexual dysfunction. The practicing alcoholic who complains of impotence is not a good candidate for penile implantation. Appropriate treatment of his alcoholism could well correct his sexual dysfunction without the need for surgery. Patients with impotence after perineal trauma should wait at least 12 to 18 months after the injury before considering themselves as irreversibly impotent.

Impotence after total prostatectomy and radical cystectomy has long been recognized as a postoperative complication. Preoperative discussion of the procedure to be carried out will usually include a frank discussion of the possibility of impotence. Most urologists would agree that this patient probably has a 99 per cent chance of being unable to achieve a satisfactory erection. In one study of 104 patients who had undergone radical prostatectomy, 23 per cent indicated that they were not impotent; they were either able to achieve penile tumescence suitable for vaginal penetration or they could gain vaginal penetration with the flaccid penis.[1] In another 15 per cent, impotence was denied because orgasm could be achieved. These patients should be carefully evaluated as to their current sex practices and their expectations of surgery.

Psychologic Evaluation. It has been stated that one of the best indications that impotence is psychogenic rather than organic is the occurrence of nocturnal and morning erections.[4] Such erections are thought to be associated with rapid eye movements during sleep. It is assumed by Karacan et al.[5] that patients who do not have nocturnal penile tumescence are organically impotent and have a poor prognosis when psychotherapy is employed. On the other hand, impotence associated with nocturnal penile tumescence is considered to have a favorable prognosis with the potential for restored potency through psychotherapy and dietary regulation. There are many patients, however, who do not respond to such treatment or are not suitable candidates for psychotherapy but who may be excellent candidates for surgical restoration of sexual function.

All patients to be considered for surgical correction should undergo psychologic testing and consultation. Psychologic screening through the use of the Minnesota Multiphasic Personality Inventory (MMPI) has been extremely helpful in our patient selection. According to Dr. David Osborne,[8] the MMPI is useful in identifying some emotional factors in impotent patients which increase susceptibility to psychogenic impotence.

Use of the penile plethysmograph has been advocated by some investigators to detect nocturnal penile tumescence and thereby distinguish organic from psychogenic impotence.[5] I have not had occasion to use this test, for I find that the MMPI, urologic review, and psychiatric interview are sufficient for distinguishing the overtly psychogenically impotent male from the one whose impotence is organically induced. In our opinion, deciding whether or not the impotence is organic is only a minor part of the workup. Our main concern is whether the patient is likely to respond to some less drastic form of treatment regardless of the basis for the impotence.

Age and Health. Surgeons who implant prosthetic devices do not consider age to be a factor in patient selection. In a recent review of penile implants involving several different types of prosthetic devices, the ages ranged from 22 to 79 years.[2,10,12] It is generally agreed that a more important factor in patient selection is the current status of the patient's health and its potential influence on the successful implantation of the prosthetic device. At the time of this writing we have not experienced a single surgical death in 132 patients receiving an implant with the inflatable penile prosthesis.

Motivation. All patients seeking surgical correction of their impotence should be carefully evaluated as to their motivation. As mentioned earlier, both man and wife should be interviewed by the physician in order that both have a clear understanding of what can be achieved through the use of sex prosthetics and how these goals are to be accomplished surgically. To this end, a demonstration of the device to the patient, and to the spouse if he is married, is in my opinion essential. Patient-partner mutual acceptance of the prosthetic device is essential if the surgeon is to fulfill the preoperative goals set forth. The patient or his partner has on occasion rejected implantations once he or she has been helped to visualize what must be done to achieve an erection.

For the purposes of preoperative evaluation, we have created a model of the human trunk, cut away to show the positioning of the prosthetic device (Fig. 1). We have found this model invaluable in discussing plans for correction of the patient's impotence.

SURGICAL TECHNIQUE IN THE TREATMENT OF MALE IMPOTENCE

The primary objective in the surgical correction of male impotence is the establishment of a rigid penis suitable for vaginal penetration and the subsequent act of sexual intercourse. A number of techniques have been set forth in an effort to achieve this goal; however, only a few have thus far received widespread acceptance among the medical profession.

238

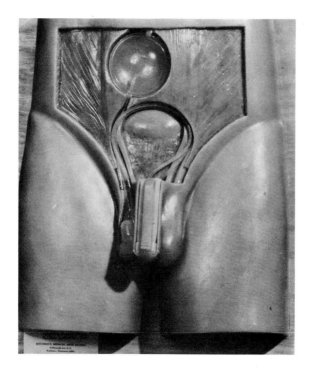

Fig. 1. Model of inflatable penile prosthesis used for demonstration purposes.

[Figs. 1 and 3 from Furlow, W.L.
Surgical management of impotence using the inflatable penile
prosthesis: experience with 36
patients. Mayo Clin. Proc.
51:325, 1976.]

The first prosthetic device to be used was the semirigid silicone rod
described by Pearman.[9] This single semirigid rod was placed beneath
Buck's fascia on the dorsum of the penis, its length tailored to fit from the
base of the penis to the corona of the glans. In essence, this technique
provided a splinting action and thereby permitted vaginal penetration.
Results with this device were fairly acceptable, although several problems occurred which were found to result in subsequent failure to achieve
satisfactory vaginal penetration. If the distal end of the rod lay behind the
corona, buckling of the glans would result and could be quite painful, as
could migration of the silicone rod laterally and ventrally. The popularity
of the device seems to have declined in the light of these reports. In
addition, the prosthesis has occasionally fractured in situ and resulted in
rather significant discomfort to the patient.[6]

A more popular modification of the semirigid rod concept is the
Small-Carrion prosthesis.[13] This prosthesis consists of two semirigid
silicone rods implanted in the corpora cavernosa of the penis which
produce a permanent semirigid penis of very satisfactory length and rigidity suitable for vaginal penetration and sexual intercourse (Fig. 2).
Proponents of this technique aptly point out the simplicity with which
the device is implanted into the penis, the absence of mechanical parts,
and the low incidence of complications.

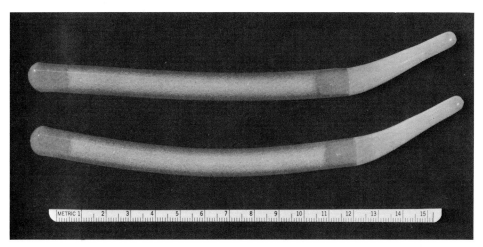

Fig. 2. Small-Carrion prosthesis. This prosthesis is available in two different diameters and in various lengths.

In a recent review of his experience with 160 Small-Carrion penile prosthetic implants, Dr. Small reported an overall complication rate of 0.5 per cent. The main problem has been accurate placement of the prosthesis with respect to length in order to avoid what has been called an "SST" deformity of the glans. The prosthesis may be implanted by the perineal approach or by dorsal incision in the midportion of the corpora. Melman[7] believes that the problem of infection is significantly minimized by the latter approach. Prolonged postoperative penile pain and penile perforation have also been reported, but these are rare complications and should not be considered specific disadvantages of the procedure. The rigidity of the rods has also been known to cause urethral erosion. Another disadvantage in the use of this prosthesis is the difficulty to be encountered if the patient subsequently requires transurethral treatment of various lower genitourinary tract problems such as bladder tumor, benign prostatic hypertrophy, and urethral strictures. Cystoscopic treatment of this type of disorder usually requires perineal urethrostomy.

Perhaps the greatest objection to the use of the Small-Carrion prosthesis is that it creates a permanent semirigid erection that may necessitate a variety of maneuvers to conceal the semierect penis underneath the clothing. Placing the penis up on the abdomen or down against the thigh has been suggested as effective. Appropriate loose clothing is sometimes necessary to conceal the penis. Very little is said about these problems in the literature, although Dr. Small has stated that in his experience the flexibility of the prosthesis is such that the phallus remains inconspicuous under various types of shorts; he does not believe that the permanent erection has deterred patients from selecting this type of prosthesis.

The inflatable penile prosthesis designed by Scott et al.[11] offers an entirely different concept in sex prosthetics for males. This hydraulically operated device consists of two expandable silicone cylinders positioned bilaterally in the corpora (Fig. 3). Each cylinder is connected to an inflate-deflate pump by tubing. The inflate-deflate pump is positioned subcutaneously in a scrotal pouch. A silicone reservoir that contains the fluid used to inflate the expandable cylinder is placed beneath the right or left rectus muscle superficially and is connected by a silicone tube to the inflate-deflate pump (Fig. 3). The entire device is implanted within the body through a small transverse suprapubic incision, thus avoiding an incisional scar in the penile or scrotal skin.

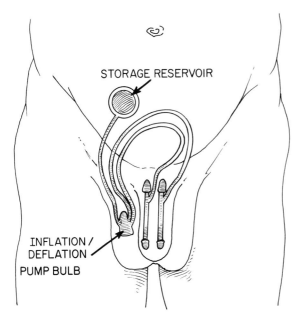

STORAGE RESERVOIR

INFLATION / DEFLATION PUMP BULB

Fig. 3. Diagram of inflatable penile prosthesis.

Activation of the inflate portion of the pump causes fluid to be pumped into the two expandable cylinders and this produces an erection similar to that normally achieved by vascular engorgement of the corpora. Once an erection is established, the penis will remain erect until the deflate portion of the pump is activated. In this manner the patient is able to maintain an erection for as long as is necessary to have satisfactory intercourse for himself and his partner. Activation of the deflate portion of the pump then allows the fluid in the cylinders to flow back into the reservoir; this causes the cylinders to deflate and the penis to become flaccid.

Urologists who have implanted this device have found it to be a highly satisfactory method of reestablishing potency. As with the Small-Carrion prosthesis, complications are minimal. In my own experience with

103 patients who have had the inflatable penile prosthesis implanted, the only significant pathologic complication has been infection (4 of 103).[3] As with other silicone prosthetic devices, it is usually necessary to remove the prosthesis if infection develops; however, once the infection has been treated and eradicated, a new prosthesis can be implanted.

Since this prosthesis is a mechanical device, it is to be expected that mechanical complications will occur. In my experience, we can expect about an 8 per cent rate of mechanical complications. These include cylinder ballooning, which may result in asymmetric penile expansion; faulty pumping mechanism; and fluid loss resulting in inadequate expansion of the cylinders. Although I have encountered all of these complications, it is important to recognize that they are correctable, although usually requiring additional surgery. These findings are comparable to the experience of others who have used the inflatable penile prosthesis.

The principal advantage of the inflatable penile prosthesis is the nearly physiologic function of this device. With this device implanted, the patient is able to have an erection when the occasion calls for it, and at other times he can maintain an inconspicuous flaccid penis suitable for the normal selection of both under and outer clothing according to his choice of fashions. The penile shaft attains a rigidity that is nearly normal to palpation, and patient-partner acceptance has been excellent. The overall functional success rate with the inflatable penile prosthesis is 95 per cent (Table 3).

Table 3. Inflatable Penile Prosthesis: Current Status of 103 Patients		
Mechanically functioning		99
Satisfactory intercourse	98	
Unsatisfactory intercourse	1	
Failure		4
Total		103

The main disadvantage of this device is that it is an artificial prosthetic device and therefore susceptible to the complications experienced with most artificially implanted devices. The mechanical nature of this device has also created some degree of physician dependence by the patient. I have not found these disadvantages to be a significant deterrent to the selection of this device by nearly all patients considered to be suitable candidates for penile implantation.

SUMMARY

Sex prosthetic devices have become an established form of therapy for both organically and psychogenically impotent males who are

242

found to be suitable candidates for this form of therapy. The techniques of implanting a penile prosthesis are well established, and the functional success with a prosthetic device approximates 90 to 95 per cent. Complications are both pathologic and mechanical and occur with relatively low frequency. I am not aware of any operative or postoperative deaths associated with the implantation of more than 5,000 devices. I believe that the availability of penile prosthetics to the impotent patient is limited only by his ability to meet the rigid criteria for patient selection. Considerations in selection include patient-partner motivation, the historical aspects of the patient's impotence, the general health of the patient, and the psychologic evaluation. If the criteria are met and it is established that the patient's expectations are in harmony with the known results provided by implantation, then we can expect uniformly successful results.

REFERENCES

1. Furlow, W.L. Personal communication.
2. ——. The current status of the inflatable penile prosthesis in the management of impotence: Mayo Clinic experience updated. J. Urol. 119:363, 1978.
3. ——. Surgical management of impotence using the inflatable penile prosthesis: experience with 103 patients. Br. J. Urol. (In press)
4. Karacan, I. Clinical value of nocturnal erection in the progress and diagnosis of impotence. Med. Aspects Hum. Sexuality 4:27, 1970.
5. Karacan, I., Williams, R.L. et al. Sleep-related penile tumescence as a function of age. Am. J. Psychiat. 132:932, 1976.
6. Mandler, J. Personal communication.
7. Melman, A. Experience with implantation of the Small-Carrion penile implant for organic impotence. J. Urol. 116:49, 1976.
8. Osborne, D. Psychologic evaluation of impotent men. Mayo Clin. Proc. 51:363, 1976.
9. Pearman, R.O. Treatment of organic impotence by implantation of a penile prosthesis. J. Urol. 97:716, 1976.
10. Raz, S. and Kaufman, J.J. Small-Carrion operation for impotence: improved technique. Urology 7:68, 1976.
11. Scott, F.B., Bradley, W.E. and Timm, G.W. Management of erectile impotence: use of implantable inflatable prosthesis. Urology 2:80, 1973.
12. Small, M.P. Small-Carrion penile prosthesis: a report on 160 cases and review of the literature. J. Urol. 119:365, 1978.
13. Small, M.P., Carrion, H.M. and Gordon, J.A. Small-Carrion penile prosthesis: new implant for management of impotence. Urology 5:479, 1975.

20

Sex Education of Children
with Disabilities

MARGARET E. SYMONDS, M.D., LORAINE WICKWARE, R.N.

Sex education for disabled children should begin at the same time as sexual activity—at birth. Just as the erotogenic areas can be stimulated in the infant, so may his psyche receive sexual messages, for better or for worse. These emotional effects are produced primarily by his immediate caretakers, usually his parents. By far the most significant factor affecting an individual's sex life in the fullest meaning of the term is the impression he receives from his parents. The attitude the parents give him of sexuality (companionship, intimacy, child-bearing and raising) and even more important, of their feelings regarding himself, is the material with which he builds his own sexual jigsaw puzzle. Thus the physician's task when confronted with a newborn infant with disfiguring or disabling defects, or when disease or accident occurs to an older child, is to help the parents accept the child and adjust to the defects.

Helping the parents accept the child and his problems is no magic wand-waving task for the physician, but a careful, inverted pyramid structure, beginning with the moment he first tells them about the child, helps them and comforts them as they pass through grief (bereavement for the perfect child they expected), disbelief (denial) and anger, and guides them through together to acceptance. Of course it is not all up to the physician—he has to bring to the parents' aid the next expanding layer of the pyramid, the obstetric and pediatric nursing and social service teams. His task will be a much more hopeful one if the parents have a "good" marriage, are generous and mutually supporting, and if they love children as children and not as (potential) fulfillers of their ambitions.

The parents will need to do a good deal of mutual supporting through dark, anxious days, with vacations omitted, luxuries gone without, and leisure time given over to journeys to hospitals, nights at the sick bed, and hours spent teaching the handicapped child skills such as walking and talking that a normal child learns naturally by himself.

The physician must stay with the parents during the first hours of shock and grief, into the learning process (parents must learn to be therapists) and through the struggle to obtain all the needed services for the child. The base of the inverted pyramid, spreading upward from this apex at the bottom, is formed by all the rehabilitation team members, the school teachers, friends and citizens of the world that shape the child's life from without. If the physician who first breaks the news then stays with the child and his parents, guiding them, finding answers to almost insoluble problems, and comforting them with the sure knowledge that all that can be done is being done, to the point where the child can face the future independent of his parents and be ready to enter the adult world, he is indeed a friend of the family. This kind of support enables the parents to persevere, gives them the resourcefulness to stay together in harmony, and mutually love their child. Without this love, the child cannot love himself, cannot see himself as a worthy love-object, and will lack the generosity to love another. Thus it is the cornerstone of a child's sex education.

All other aspects of sex education follow along exactly the same line as for "normal children." His genital exploration and play need the same degree of acceptance and he needs to be taught "time and place," socially acceptable behavior and restraint without repression. The physician must realize, and guide the parents accordingly, that most people have feelings somewhat akin to aversion to the idea of "cripples" and "freaks" having normal sexual feelings, least of all enjoying sexual activity. The parents may have the same "hang-ups" and the physician (or professional counselor) must anticipate the problem and bring it into the open during the child's very early months and challenge the parents. Parents of "normal" children reveal their expectations that the child will one day himself be a parent in countless ways. "When you are grown up and have children of your own," or "now you have outgrown that book, it can stay on your shelf and one day you will be able to read it to your little girl," and so on. By such means the parents assign the role, and the child absorbs it along with his daily bread and ABCs.

The parent must be taught to answer truthfully the child's sexual questions, so the physician must ensure that the parent is herself correctly informed. The genetics of the disorder, necessary knowledge for the parents' future family planning, should also be discussed from the point of view of the child's reproductive future. If the genetic pattern, or the nature of the condition itself, precludes the desirability of reproduction, this should be discussed with the parent and the child made aware of it at a reasonably early age, well before the onset of puberty. The parents should be helped to discuss the situation frequently with the physician and with each other, so that they are better able to be matter-of-fact in their presentation of the idea to the child. Such statements as "when you grow up, you can adopt a little orphan so that he does not come with legs/back/heart like yours and have to have all the same nasty operations and days in the hospital that you have had," can be used to plant the idea in the receptive soil of the young child's mind.

As the child grows older and reaches school age, his next real teachers of the "facts of life" are his peers—they are the agents that modify (again for better or for worse) the child's opinion of himself. Try as they will, parents and physicians can do little to control the words and actions of the kids at school or in the neighborhood. All they can do is help the child accept comments and questions with good grace, helped by both words of advice, and by their own continued loving acceptance. It is better to have children from outside the family meet the child with a disability on his own home ground. Mother and father should go out of their way to make their child's home the entertainment center for the gang. Children automatically like to play where the parents provide a warm, happy and exciting atmosphere and this ensures companions for the child whose lack of ambulation ties him to the house or to sedentary activities.

Not only does peer group interaction slowly and insensibly (but let us hope not too insensitively) add a new dimension to a child's self-image, but sex talk and exchange of information (frequently wildly off-target) is a necessary part of his sex education.

The time comes when the physician or other professional is usually the best person to sit down with the child and let him ask questions, air fears that are bothering him and learn about his own sexual function. This is best brought about in the course of a "routine" office or hospital visit when the child is nearing sexual maturation.

If the parent feels able to deal with this, and is fully informed by the physician, so much the better; but the young person must have the opportunity to learn and inquire. Frequently, a series of such discussions is needed, since more questions arise as some are answered. Recently the writer broached the subject with a 15-year-old paraplegic girl—in the course of a routine back examination—by first of all admiring her clothes. (This led to a discussion of the fact that her close buddy, two years older than herself, was a model in a teen department of a store and bought the clothes she modeled for her at a huge discount.) I then said, "You are lucky to be so slim; but you may be almost too slim when it comes to having babies and may need to have them delivered by cesarian section." My luck held and Dawn said, "Yes, my mother always had a cesarian because she is so small." At the next visit Dawn, who obviously had been thinking about my comments, asked about her future sex life, and we sat down and talked the thing through comfortably and completely.

Contraception these days is not a big issue; all the kids know where they are with it, and how to obtain adequate care. But children with sensory deficits and even more so those with enterostomies or abnormal genitalia need to be informed about alternative methods of intercourse, non-genital erotogenic areas and all the "other options" open to "normal," as well as disabled persons. It is necessary to be explicit here, to produce diagrams and appropriate literature to help in these explanations.

The time of approaching sexual maturity is the time when genetics and other pros and cons of childbearing should be gently brought to the handicapped young person's attention. As in any genetic counseling situation, the truthful, unembellished facts should be offered in a form that can be understood. The individual herself must then decide how to use the knowledge, and whether to attempt to produce children or not.

Perhaps the final advice the parents or other caretakers of young people with disabilities need to be given is the most difficult for them to accept— and that is, to allow the boys and girls the necessary privacy for petting and sexual experimentation. Ground rules cannot be laid down for this aspect of the problem—each situation must be managed according to the circumstances, the degree of sexual permissiveness of the parents and the degree of maturity and independence of the "partners" being paramount.

This discussion may have seemed to assume that all disabled children may be expected to grow up in benign, loving families and be able to develop good self-images, with courage and confidence enough to face the world. Needless to say, this is the exception rather than the rule. Adolescence for the disabled is almost always an even more seering, agonizing experience than for "normal" teenagers. They have only to look in the mirror, or down at their limbs and body, to know all too readily that she is not Olga Korbut or he is not Rudolph Nureyev. Rejection by parents, siblings or peers somewhere along the line has occurred, academic or athletic failure has been experienced. Here again, early education, beginning with education of the parents, can in part forestall this problem. More than any other, the disabled individual must be taught to contribute to others' welfare—whether by acquiring skills to earn a good living, or by becoming a good cook, or by learning to contribute to people's social pleasures, being a good listener or a good raconteur. (I once enjoyed a rush-hour traffic jam in the Lincoln Tunnel while a paraplegic friend entertained me with an animated account of how she and several of her fellow patients at the Hospital for Special Surgery's School, sneaked out to light a candle—though none of them was a Catholic, or knew how to perform such a task—for a parentless friend who was about to undergo major surgery.) Love, affection and deep mutual regard are, after all, more enduring aphrodisiacs than is physical perfection.

Perhaps the biggest step forward in the field of sex education of the handicapped will have been made when the population at large—physicians, other professionals, parents, all people in general—realize that being disfigured or crippled or retarded does not of itself abolish the desire for love and its sexual expression, and that adult men and women are entitled to the joy of it, quite as much as everyone else. There is nothing wrong about being cerebral palsied, or retarded, or blind...and in love. What is wrong is to keep apart two people who together could face the world better than could each alone.

21

Sexuality in the Institutionalized
Patient

ALEX COMFORT, M.B.

People who suffer from certain disabilities may be obliged to live in an institutional setting. In doing so they surrender privacy and autonomy to an institutional staff. While in the general world most people escape from the overt standards of society, or can do so if they wish, the institution is bound to act those standards out. Very often it does so with a time-lag of many years interposed between the lifestyle of the general community and the preconceptions which institutional living upholds. Inpatients were formerly forcibly restrained from masturbation: although masturbation is now accepted by most individuals as a component of normal sexuality, and many institutional staffs are advised not to notice it, there is a quantitative gap between this kind of blind-eye-turning and the positive provision of privacy. Institutions may be, and often are, one-sex in composition; are they prepared to accept rather than overlook homosexual outlets? More threatening still, are they prepared to facilitate heterosexual expression, and if so, how?

These are problems which we normally handle by overlooking them in the hope that they will go away. Yet even if we ignore "community standards," it is extraordinarily hard to devise even in theory a humane, responsible and viable solution which recognizes need and develops human dignity. What sexual mercy is shown in these settings is probably incidental and spontaneous, and the policy of overlooking rather than organizing has a lot to be said for it. With humane and sexually positive staffs (which are becoming commoner) this policy might work better than controversial experiment. On the other hand, the chief sexual problem of the institutionalized disabled is the projected anxiety, embarrassment and unease of the staff—arising mostly from not knowing anything to say or do which might be helpful. In this area, the Sexual Attitude Reassessment Program (SAR) for staff—or better for staff and patients together—can do a lot to discharge the anxieties of both and to enable the narrow-minded Nurse Ratchetts of this world to reassess or move on. The problem will have to be met; it is a microcosm of the discrepancy between action and legislation, between what we do and what we profess, which produces so much irrationality and friction at all the points where individual behaviors and public attitudes meet.

The arguments in favor of encouraging or actively providing sexual activity for longterm institutionalized patients, even if that activity is somewhat impersonal, are that many patients would welcome it, already fantasize about it, and would have their confined world enriched by it. Knowing oneself to be sexually functional is an immense ego reinforcement; the large moral emphasis on the personal and relational as the only valid sexual mode is itself a culture-based fantasy, bearing little relation to the way sex is normally used in much modern living. There is something slightly idiotic in directing the physiotherapist who observes sexual response during whole-body massage to put a towel over it and pretend it is not there. A person incapable of masturbation will never experience waking orgasm unless assisted.

The counter-arguments center on imagined (and sometimes validly imagined) problems: whether it is humane to "turn on" those whose opportunities will be limited (on the assumption that none of them is spontaneously "turned on" already); whether satisfaction once humanely afforded will become a demand; whether sexual servicing will be experienced (especially by women) as demeaning to the recipient, and who is to administer the service? A relatively unexploited resource in answering some of these quite well-taken questions might be to ask the persons concerned, a method rarely used with hospital patients and very rarely with the disabled, around whom a whole institutional dynamic of social incompetence and "childrenization" has often been created.

The increasing outside acceptance of sexuality as potentially a social or friendly as well as a reproductive or relational gesture may affect this argument in time, but social changes penetrate institutions slowly through the nature of institutions themselves and of institutionists. The advocates of change certainly recognize that where the relational is at all possible it must take precedence; at this level, for example, homosexual relational sex, even between those who would by inclination prefer heterosexual, can be personally enriching. On the other hand, for many disabled persons, the emphasis on our culture's conventional view of relational sex is unhelpful simply for lack of realistic opportunity, and even if it is not, self-trial as a sexual person may be needed to generate the energy to create or pursue opportunity. "Disabled people" differ here quite as much as the able. Some want no part of, or are embarrassed by, the possibility of sexual expression. Quite a number recognize and would enjoy without guilt or soul-searching its recreational and experiential potential, just as they would enjoy a ride in a car. Being more chronically exposed than we are to having their choices made for them by others who "know better," they may have to show considerable stamina in order to be asked what they personally would appreciate. Accordingly, the first step in planning any opening up of institutions to sex is *full discussion,* not between able experts about what would be good for their patients, but between and with patients about what they would like or dislike. The task of the staff is to control their own projected anxieties and to avoid impertinent or voyeuristic zeal and the creation of imaginary dangers.

If the reaction of patients is positive, patients and staff must then discuss who is to provide what is being asked for (the very idea of such discussion might render some superintendents apoplectic; it should be led by someone skilled in group therapy who could deal with unextinguished fuses at the end of the session). Such a discussion often tends toward the view that the regular staff, whose interaction with patients is already structured, are not the best people to undertake an additional and potentially disturbing role. Most of the risks which might reasonably be foreseen with the introduction of sexual contacts are really exaggerations of the problems of any longterm institutional relationship—jealousy, exploitation, "crushes," and dependency. The professional status of the staff provides a measure of protective clothing which their patients value—after all, in the hospital one has to live with the staff, and one needs to avoid unnecessary tensions since unlike the outside world, a hospital affords no equivalent of leaving town.

Patients tend to find security in this distancing, and staff still more so. Though not strictly enforceable, it is a barrier which spontaneous acts of sexual kindness and concern, like other acts of kindness and concern, rightly cross. Overzealous prohibition for fear that these feelings may prove misconceived increases the body-image problems of the severely disabled person who cannot touch others, and whom others have been told not to touch with concern for fear of being misunderstood. Legislation here is no substitute for common sense: after all, staff members and patients may fall in love and marry with full conventional honors. By general professional consent, physicians and nurses should not become sexually involved with patients in their care except in the conventionally approved context, and the reasons against any dilution of this principle are overwhelming—all patients require the presence of individuals who retain a specifically nonsexual role. In some Scandinavian institutions, the persons most involved have been physiotherapists. One can imagine the effects of any heavyhanded attempt to institutionalize this situation. The alternative is the concerned visitor; where the patient has personal friends of the opposite sex, most hospitals would not find it intolerable at least to provide privacy. As to those who have no such friends, one may recall the situation in Britain during World War II, when airmen with severe facial burns were informally provided with female escorts who helped them overcome both their fear of appearing in public and their fear of rejection through disfigurement. What was then a humane and patriotic relationship is harder to translate informally in the context of lifelong institutional deprivation, but it should not be beyond the wit of man.

Although institutions in Scandinavia and elsewhere have addressed this difficult problem, the lack of published references speaks to the good sense of the persons and institutions involved. The two most serious barriers to the working-out of humane and commonsense solutions are likely to be publicity and attempted organization. There is probably no more suitable field for the privacy of doctor-patient communication.

The sexual visitor would have a difficult task. He or she must basically be the initiator, so that nobody is disappointed, but unobvious, so that the transaction is not perfunctory, and above all totally unembarrassed. Massage, as in outside life, is a good icebreaker, and the transition can be unspoken or asked ("Do you want me to go on?"). Sexual experience is also essential, if only to provide the feedback necessary to satisfy a partner who cannot provide all the usual cues, and with whom a failure of any kind is to be avoided at all costs.

There is no category of persons who possess these skills unless we create one, although more people now have them than in the recent past. Prostitutes were, and possibly still are, a resource for the male disabled. As a class, with exceptions, they make poor training partners for able people with functional sexual problems because their choice of occupation quite often covers a basic dislike of the opposite sex, and their normal pattern may emphasize speed of performance. With the disabled, however, they often perform very much better and with genuine concern, since the client poses no unconscious threat. Professional surrogates, a recent development in the United States, are also very often women who relate particularly well to dysfunctional males (the number of male surrogates is as yet too small for any profile to be drawn). A serious program to introduce sex into institutions could not be based on either of these categories. It would be much better based on

personal recruitment of concerned men and women having the necessary qualifications by members of the staff who pass the word privately
among the sexually unembarrassed. As in all other matters touching the
sexual relations of people, publicity of every kind should be avoided
and privacy safeguarded, by total denial if necessary. Interference by
the righteous is best met by suggesting that their moral sensitivity be
redirected to topics more wholesome for society than the officious per-
secution of the disabled.

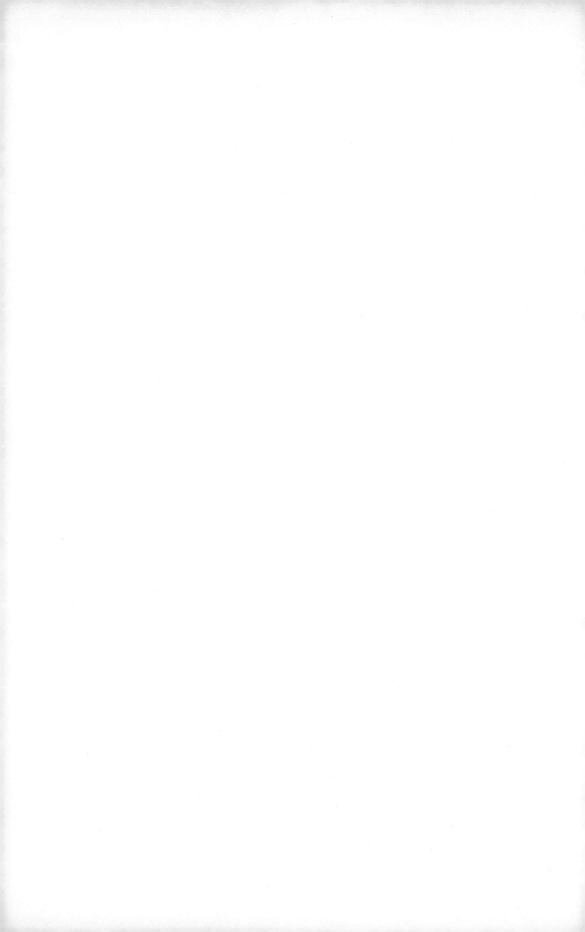

22

Sexual Attitude Reassessment Programs, Rehabilitation Professionals and the Physically Disabled

LAURO S. HALSTEAD, M.D.

SECTION 1: **An Interdisciplinary Program on Human Sexuality for Health Care Professionals and the Physically Disabled: Rationale and Description**

Rationale

The problem of sexuality in medicine has been widely neglected in the past because patients and professionals alike generally find it a topic with which they are ill at ease. This is especially true in persons with longterm physical disabilities as pointed out by Weiss and Diamond[1] in patients with myelopathy, by Richardson[2] in persons with cerebral palsy and by Cole[3] and others in those with spinal cord injuries. As a result, problems of sexuality are frequently undiagnosed, mismanaged or simply ignored. In order to provide appropriate treatment, counseling and support, it is necessary that a professional be comfortable with his or her own sexuality so that inhibitory and prohibitive attitudes are not conveyed which might hinder the patient's efforts toward sexual adjustment.

One of the most effective techniques for helping people reevaluate their personal and professional feelings regarding sexuality is the Sexual Attitude Reassessment (SAR) Program originally developed by the National Sex and Drug Forum in San Francisco[4] and later modified at the University of Minnesota for use with medical students, spinal cord injured adults and health care professionals.[5,6] These programs have now been widely imitated and adopted in many centers around the country. In April 1973, a 2½-day workshop based on the pioneering programs in San Francisco and Minnesota was initiated at the Texas Institute for Rehabilitation and Research (TIRR).[7] Although reassessment of personal sexual attitudes has been the primary goal of this program, several closely related objectives have emerged: 1) evaluate the impact of the workshop on changing both sexual attitudes and behaviors; 2) evaluate the sexual satisfaction and problem areas of participants with particular reference to persons with physical disabilities; and 3) provide an institute-wide catalyst for initiating programs and services based on newly identified unmet needs.

PROGRAM DESCRIPTION

TIRR is an 81-bed rehabilitation facility within the Texas Medical Center in Houston. It is a private, not-for-profit hospital affiliated with Baylor College of Medicine. Since April 1973, TIRR has sponsored 18 SAR workshops. Although there have been variations from program to program, the basic objectives and format have remained essentially the same. The major objective was to help participants reassess their sexual attitudes and assist them in becoming more comfortable with their own sexuality both personally and professionally. The assumptions which underlie the philosophy of the workshop and the program objectives are listed in Tables 1 and 2. Both the assumptions and objectives are revised and adapted from the program at the University of Minnesota.

Table 1. Assumptions.

1. Sex is a health issue and most of us, both disabled and able-bodied, have sexual problems at one time or another.
2. We need more than our own personal experience and private opinions to find the best answers to sexual problems.
3. Our ability to solve sexual problems is often handicapped by our personal taboos, biases and overreactions.
4. Health professionals who have useful information concerning sexual problems often lack the ability or comfort to use the information they have.
5. Physically disabled people have much to contribute to the sexual adjustment of others because they often have had to deal directly with their own.

Table 2. Objectives.

1. To provide a comfortable and safe setting to discuss one's feelings about sexuality.
2. To help bring anxieties regarding sexuality to the surface so that they can be better understood.
3. To increase understanding of one's own attitudes and sexuality in order to accept one's self and deal more effectively with others.
4. To increase tolerance of the wide variety of human sexual behaviors and responses.
5. To understand the physically disabled person's sexual attitudes and behaviors.
6. To foster the recognition that we are all sexual people whether professional or non-professional, disabled or able-bodied, and to initiate discussion, as equals, of this aspect of our lives.
7. To make sexuality as enjoyable as possible.

While the objectives are clearly stated, it is equally important to indicate what the program is *not*. Specifically, it is not a series of lectures or didactic sessions; while some factual material is presented, the major emphasis is on the attitudinal aspects of sexuality. It is not therapy, an encounter session, or a T-group. Participants are not required to do or say anything which would cause them embarrassment or make them uncomfortable.

The 2½-day workshop uses a multimedia presentation to cover a wide variety of topics. Films, tapes, slides, talks and small group discussions are used in dealing directly and explicitly with a wide variety of sexual activities. At strategic points throughout the workshop, participants meet in small groups of 10 to 12 persons with trained leaders to examine and share materials and topics presented. An outline of the topics and methods of presentation is described for each day in Table 3.

Pre- and post-workshop attitudes regarding various sexual activities were obtained using a modification of the Minnesota Sexual Attitude Scales (MSAS). The MSAS is shown in Table 4 and contains nine scales describing nine different sexual activities which range from the use of fantasy to stimulate private masturbation to engaging in group sex. Participants were asked to describe how they felt about each of the nine sexual activities on a scale from 1 to 5 where 1 equals "I feel great about it" to 5 which equals "I feel repulsed by it." Participants also completed anonymous questionnaires concerning their experiences and satisfaction with specific sexual behaviors. In addition, they were asked to describe their level of sexual activity during the six months preceding the workshop and the reasons for any decrease in the desired level of sexual activity. The stability of attitude changes was evaluated through fol-

Table 3. Program description.

Topic	Presentation
Day 1: Friday 6:30 p.m.–10:30 p.m.	
Pre-workshop evaluation	Questionnaire (sexual attitudes, behavior & satisfaction)
Universality of sex	Art slides
Explicit words	Filmstrips
Fantasy	Film
Nudity	Film
Masturbation	Historical readings; films
Small Group Discussion	
Day 2: Saturday 8:30 a.m.–5:00 p.m.	
Desensitization (Pornography)	Commercial films
Resensitization:	
Sexuality in the context of caring relationships	
Heterosexuality	Films: able-bodied and disabled
Homosexuality	Films; gay panel
Communication and sex roles	Readings; skit; tape
3 Small Group Discussions	
Day 3: Sunday 8:30 a.m.–4:00 p.m.	
Sexological examination	Film
Sex without intercourse	Tape
Sexuality in the physically disabled	Patient panel
Spinal cord injury, cerebral palsy	Films
Sexuality and health care: Evaluation, Diagnosis, Counseling, Treatment, etc.	Interdisciplinary panel
2 Small Group Discussions	
Post-workshop evaluation	Questionnaire (program content and sexual attitudes)

low-up questionnaires mailed to participants approximately six months following their workshop experience. In addition, participants were asked to evaluate the general value of the workshop and its impact on changing their personal sexual satisfaction. These results are described in Section II.

From the beginning, the TIRR program has been a low-budget, largely self-supporting effort. Tuition for the first program was $2.50 and all staff participation was on a volunteer basis. Although we have been forced to raise the tuition to meet necessary costs and purchase our own films and equipment, freely contributed time and effort by staff

Table 4. Minnesota Sexual Attitude Scales (MSAS).

I.	Using erotica (erotic literature, pictures, films, live sex shows, etc.) to stimulate sexual arousal.
II.	Fantasy as a sexual stimulant in private masturbation.
III.	Mutual masturbation with someone of the opposite sex.
IV.	Mutual masturbation with someone of the same sex.
V.	Sexual intercourse with someone of the opposite sex.
VI.	Oral-genital stimulation with someone of the opposite sex.
VII.	Oral-genital stimulation with someone of the same sex.
VIII.	Engaging in sex with your partner in the presence of others.
IX.	Three or more people engaging in intercourse and other sexual activity together.

members from all disciplines still play an important role in helping to minimize overall expenses. Table 5 shows a summary of expenses for an average workshop during 1975. For 50 participants, the total cost is

Table 5. Summary of Workshop Expenses (1975)

Core Staff	$600.00
Group Leaders	400.00
Food	350.00
Film purchase and replacement	200.00
Patient Panel	175.00
Printing	100.00
Gay Panel	75.00
Audio-visual equipment management	75.00
Film rental	75.00
Mail/printing	50.00
Contingence/miscellaneous	200.00
	$2,300.00
Participants	50
Cost per participant	$46.00

approximately $2300 or $46 per participant. Actual tuition ranges from $25 to $65 depending on ability to pay. Tuition includes four meals, a social hour and 20 hours of intensive workshop experience.

The largest expense items are for core staff, small group leaders and panel members who are reimbursed for personal expenses and investment of a significant commitment of time and effort over an entire weekend. Food and expenses associated with the audiovisual component of the program are the next largest items.

Table 6 shows the sources of payment for 609 participants. Four hundred and twenty-six or 70 per cent paid their own tuition and 14 per cent were sponsored by various educational programs. Only a small number of participants (97, or 16%) were sponsored by local health agencies, insurance companies or the vocational rehabilitation agency. Expressed in other terms, only 16 per cent were able to attend the program as an accepted, reimbursable health care service. Reasons for this low figure are the tuition fee and the fact that sexual adjustment and fulfillment—unlike most other aspects of living—are not seen as an essential or even important component of comprehensive health care by many people.

Table 6. Sources Of Payment For 609 Participants.

Sponsor	No.	%
Self-pay	426	70
Educational funds	86	14
Local agencies*	53	9
Insurance	32	5
Vocational Rehabilitation Agency	12	2
Total	609	100

*Multiple Sclerosis, Muscular Dystrophy, Cerebral Palsy, Visiting Nurse Association.

Over the past four years the program has undergone significant changes in many areas which are described in more detail elsewhere.[8] In brief, however, the program initially was made available exclusively for patients and staff associated with TIRR. Gradually as this population group was covered, it became clear that the same program was equally adaptable to other disability groups. Initially, it was also felt desirable to separate workshops for the staff and those for patients. However, with experience it became evident that the problems were essentially identical for both groups, and that furthermore, it was a much richer experience when staff, patients and students were allowed to mix and learn from each other. The same has been true with regard to mixing patients with various disabilities.

At present, anyone may attend from within the medical or lay communities. The only restriction is that a participant must be 18 years of age or older. As we continue to expand, it is our expectation that the program will be seen as an important growth experience for an ever widening group of people. We are hoping to make it available on a regular basis as part of the medical school curriculum and we are beginning to receive referrals from local psychiatrists, ministers and marriage counselors who view the program as a good way to initiate ongoing counseling and therapy for specific sexual problems.

SECTION II: **Participant Response to SAR Workshops**

During the period from April 1973 to February 1977, the Institute has sponsored 16 SAR Workshops with 707 participants, for an average of 44 persons per program. Fifty-four per cent were women, fifty-one per cent were over 27 years of age, and 65 per cent were health care students or professionals. Five hundred and ninety-nine or 85 per cent were able-bodied, and 108 or 15 per cent of the participants had a physical disability. Of those with disabilities, the largest category (75%) had spinal cord injury. Other disability groups included multiple sclerosis, stroke, muscular dystrophy, visual impairment and cerebral palsy. For 93 per cent of the participants, this was the first workshop in human sexuality they had ever attended. Composite analysis of all post-workshop evaluations indicate that 98 per cent of the participants said they would recommend the program to others and 97 per cent felt the workshops were beneficial. Ninety-one per cent said they could discuss sex more freely as a result of attending the workshops. Finally, 97 per cent felt the workshop accomplished the goal of dispelling myths about sex, and 88 per cent expressed the opinion that this type of program should be a required part of professional training. Of the medical students who attended, 100 per cent felt this should either be an elective or a required part of the medical curriculum.

In addition to the program evaluations, sexual attitudes were measured using a modification of the Minnesota Sexual Attitude Scales (MSAS) (see Table 4). The MSAS is administered pre- and post-workshop and at 6-month intervals in followup. Pre- and post-workshop responses for 206 participants from Workshops 6 through 11 are shown in Table 7. Scales are ranked according to the size of change in pre- and post-workshop mean scores. These data reveal two major conclusions: 1) the mean scores for all nine scales were lower after the workshop— that is, the participants felt more comfortable about each of the nine sexual activities; and 2) the size of the attitudinal change for six of the nine scales was statistically significant at the 0.01 or 0.05 level using student's "t" test. These six scales refer to the following activities: using fantasy in private masturbation (II),* using erotic material to stimulate sexual arousal (I), oral-genital stimulation with someone of the opposite sex (VI), mutual masturbation with someone of the same sex (IV), mutual masturbation with someone of the opposite sex (III), and intercourse with someone of the opposite sex (V). The three scales which did not show a significant change in attitude among the participants refer to the following activities: oral-genital stimulation with someone of the

---

*Roman numerals refer to items in the Minnesota Sexual Attitude Scale.

Table 7. Mean Values For Pre- And Post-Workshop Responses To Sexual
Attitude Scales For 206 Participants

| Rank | Scale[1] | Mean Scores | | Change |
		Pre-Workshop	Post-Workshop	
1	II	2.04	1.59	-0.45^2
2	I	2.11	1.74	-0.37^2
3	VI	1.85	1.52	-0.33^2
4	IV	3.96	3.68	-0.28^3
5	III	1.82	1.55	-0.27^2
6	VII	4.11	3.87	-0.24
7	V	1.46	1.30	-0.16^3
8	IX	3.92	3.80	-0.12
9	VIII	4.03	3.91	-0.12

[1]Scales refer to sexual activities which are described in Table 4.
 Response code: from 1 = I feel great about it; to 5 = I feel repulsed by it.
[2]$p < 0.01$
[3]$p < 0.05$

same sex (VII), three or more people engaging in sexual activity together
(IX), and engaging in sex in the presence of others (VIII). In general, the
results reflect the kinds of changes one might expect: the larger changes
occurring with less anxiety-provoking and thus more acceptable areas
such as using fantasy and erotic materials to stimulate arousal, and the
smallest changes occurring with activities that are still somewhat taboo
and therefore more anxiety-provoking such as group sex. In a control
study of the MSAS, Held et al. reported no statistically significant
changes in a group of 18 first-year medical students who did not attend
a SAR Workshop.[9] These students were 18 to 35 years of age, and 72 per
cent were men.

The results reported here reveal a number of similarities with data
recorded by other workers using the SAR method. In the area of attitude
change, we have consistently found participants feel more comfortable
regarding various sexual activities *after* attending a SAR Workshop.
Using the original version of the MSAS in which participants were asked
to rate each activity for 5 categories of people (themselves, mid-adoles-
cents, unmarried adults, married adults, and married adults having a
secret affair), Held[9] reported on a group of 48 rehabilitation professionals
who felt more comfortable six weeks post-workshop with all nine sexual
behaviors tested, with a significant change in four of the behaviors. In a
modified form of the MSAS in which participants were asked to rate
each activity for only 2 categories of people (themselves and others), we
also found that participants—professionals, non-professionals and pa-

tients alike—felt more comfortable with all nine behaviors immediately after attending a workshop, and a significant change was noted in six of these behaviors. General post-workshop evaluations show other similarities. The percentages of participants who said our workshops were enjoyable, non-harmful and personally and professionally beneficial are approximately the same as the figures reported for the San Francisco and Minnesota programs.[4,9] Such findings are important for several reasons. One, it helps confirm the basic value and effectiveness of the SAR concept and two, it provides tangible evidence that the original workshops represent realistic models that can be adapted, transplanted and flourish under quite different circumstances.

SECTION III: **Comparison of Sexual Attitudes, Behavior and Satisfaction for Able-Bodied and Disabled Participants Attending SAR Workshops**

Pre- and post-workshop sexual attitude changes by physical status of 380 participants at Workshops 7 through 15 are shown in Table 8. For

Table 8. Pre- And Post-Workshop Sexual Attitude Changes By Physical Status For 380 Participants

Scale	Behavior	Pre- and Post-Workshop Changes[1]	
		Able (N = 321)	Disabled (N = 59)
I	Erotica for arousal	-5.49^5	-0.41
II	Masturbation	-4.97^5	-2.80^3
III	Heterosexual masturbation	-4.76^5	-2.66^3
IV	Homosexual masturbation	-4.16^5	-0.34
V	Intercourse	-3.15^4	-1.60^2
VI	Heterosexual oral-genital stimulation	-3.46^4	-2.02^2
VII	Homosexual oral-genital stimulation	-2.89^4	-1.09
VIII	Sex in presence of others	-3.55^4	-0.46
IX	Group sex	-1.07	-0.07

[1]Expressed as z scores. Significance tested using Wilcoxon's signed ranks test.
[2]$p < 0.05$ (initial criteria level)
[3]$p < 0.01$
[4]$p < 0.001$
[5]$p < 0.0001$

all nine scales, the ratings were lower following the workshop experience for both the able-bodied and disabled groups suggesting that participants felt more comfortable about each of the nine sexual activities. Among the 321 able-bodied participants, the amount of change for eight of the nine scales was statistically significant at the 0.001 or 0.0001 level using Wilcoxon's signed ranks test while among the 59 disabled participants the change was statistically significant at the 0.05 to 0.01 level in four of the nine scales. There were significant attitude changes common to both groups for four activities. These included fantasy as a stimulant in private masturbation (II),* heterosexual masturbation (III), intercourse (V) and heterosexual oral-genital activity(VI); for a fifth activity—group sex (IX)—there was no significant attitude change for either group of participants.

Table 9 summarizes by physical status the sexual experiences for 549 participants with regard to masturbation, intercourse and oral-genital

Table 9. Sexual Experience By Physical Status for 549 Participants

Activity (Ever Experienced)	Able-Bodied (N = 470)		Disabled (N = 79)		Totals (N = 549)	
	N	%	N	%	N	%
Masturbation	436	93	70	89	506	92
Intercourse	450	96	67	85	517	94
Oral-genital	423	90	60	76	483	88
Homosexuality*	24	16	5	23	29	17

*Able-bodied (N = 149); Disabled (N = 23)

activity. For 172 participants, there is also information regarding homosexuality. Data for this table were obtained in response to the question of whether or not the person had *ever* experienced any of the behaviors listed, regardless of when. As can be seen, with the exception of homosexuality, the percentages are fairly high for both groups ranging from 76 to 96 per cent. Also with the exception of homosexuality, the disabled population reported having less experience in all areas compared to the able-bodied group. The number reporting at least one homosexual experience represented 23 per cent of the disabled group compared with 16 per cent of the able-bodied group.

Sexual experience for the same activities during the six months prior to attending the workshop was also investigated. Results concerning masturbation, intercourse and oral-genital sex are shown in Table 10 for 560 participants by physical status. For 172 of these respondents, additional information regarding homosexuality is also shown. As one might expect, these figures are lower than the ones in the previous table for all activities in both groups. Among able-bodied participants, homosexuality was experienced by 12 per cent during the previous six months while for disabled participants the figure was 9 per cent. For the other three activities, comparisons between the two groups show

*Roman numerals refer to items in the Minnesota Sexual Attitude Scale.

Table 10. Sexual Experience By Physical Status During Past 6 Months For 560 Participants[1]

Activity	Able-Bodied (N=478)		Disabled (N=82)		Totals (N=560)	
	N	%	N	%	N	%
Masturbation	414	87	48	59	462	83
Intercourse	430	90	51	62	481	86
Oral-genital	393	82	48	59	441	79
Homosexuality[2]	18	12	2	9	20	12

[1]Experienced 1 or more times during 6 months prior to workshop.
[2]Able-bodied (N=149); Disabled (N=28)

marked differences, with the disabled participants being 25 to 30 per cent less active than their able-bodied counterparts.

In response to the question, "Are you currently as sexually active as you would like?", the majority or approximately 60 per cent of both the able-bodied and disabled participants responded in the negative. Table 11 lists sexual satisfaction by physical status for 547 participants. Two

Table 11. Sexual Satisfaction By Physical Status For 547 Participants

Active As You Would Like	Able-Bodied		Disabled		Totals	
	N	%	N	%	N	%
Yes	192	41	31	38	223	41
No	274	59	50	62	324	59
Totals	466	85	81	15	547	100

hundred and seventy-four or 59 per cent of the able-bodied group replied they were not as active as they would like to be, while 50 or 62 per cent gave the same reply among the disabled group. Table 12 shows the five

Table 12. Most Common Reasons For Decreased Sexual Activity By Physical Status For 401 Participants

Reasons	Able-Bodied (N=342)		Reasons	Disabled (N=59)	
	Times Cited	%		Times Cited	%
*Lack of Partners	120	35	*Lack of Partners	34	58
*Lack of Interest[1]	100	29	Not Desirable	22	37
*Communication	79	23	Physical Problems	21	36
Non-Sex Problems	74	22	*Lack of Interest[1]	14	24
Ideas Re Sex Differ from Partner's	61	18	*Communication	10	17

*Item appears in both groups.
[1]On part of respondent and/or partner.

most common reasons for decreased sexual activity by physical status for 401 participants. For both groups, "lack of partners" was cited most frequently—by 35 per cent of the able-bodied and by 58 per cent of the disabled participants. "Lack of interest" on the part of the respondent and/or partner (mentioned by 29%) and "communication problems" (23%) were the next most common reasons in the able-bodied group; the same reasons were also among the top five in the disabled group (cited by 24% and 17% respectively). The other two reasons mentioned by the able-bodied participants included "non-sex problems" (22%) and "ideas regarding sex differ from partner's" (18%). Among disabled participants, the other two reasons cited most commonly included "feelings of not being sexually desirable" (37%) and "physical problems" such as pain, impotence, weakness, spasticity, etc. (36%). Taken together the last two reasons were mentioned by approximately three-quarters of the disabled group and provide a rough indication of the impact of physical handicaps on the level of sexual dissatisfaction.

With regard to follow-up data, questionnaires mailed six months after an SAR experience were sent to 330 participants who attended 8 consecutive workshops. One hundred and sixty-four questionnaires were returned, for a response rate of 50 per cent. Participants who returned the questionnaire were slightly older and included 3 per cent more females than in the total population, while the physical status ratio was essentially the same as in the entire group. Based on these replies, 98 per cent said they still felt attending the workshop was worthwhile. Table 13 shows this group's assessment of the impact of

Table 13. Results Of 6-Month Follow-Up Impact On Sexual Satisfaction

	N	%
	(N = 164)	
Better	84	51.2
Same	79	48.2
Worse	1	0.6
Total	164	100.0

the workshop on their sexual satisfaction in the intervening six months. Fifty-one per cent felt it was better, 48 per cent felt it was the same and one person felt it was worse. Analysis by physical status showed comparable responses for both the disabled and able-bodied groups. Finally, pre-workshop and 6-month follow-up sexual attitudes were measured using the modified MSAS. Results are available for only 97 participants from four workshops. In the attitudes measured, there was a statistically significant difference at the 0.05 level or greater in 5 of the

9 scales. These refer to heterosexual and homosexual masturbation (III and IV), intercourse (V) and heterosexual and homosexual oral-genital sex (VI and VII). This compares with significant changes found in all scales for all participants in the pre- and post-workshop data except scale IX which refers to group sex. Follow-up data concerning attitude change by physical status are not yet available because the number of respondents is too small.

COMMENT

The results reported here represent the accumulated experience with an SAR program over a 4-year period. Because the SAR workshops have been open to disabled and able-bodied persons alike, they have presented a unique opportunity to compare these two groups with regard to a number of sexual areas. In reviewing these results, however, it is important to bear in mind some of the limitations inherent in the data. First, the term "disabled" refers to a heterogeneous population of handicapped persons. As Cole[10] has pointed out, the experience and problems of different disability groups vary widely, and to treat them as if they were a homogeneous population is misleading. The specific disabilities involved in this study cover a broad spectrum which includes congenital and acquired lesions as well as relatively stable and progressive disorders. Because the total number of disabled persons available for study was relatively small, no attempt was made to analyze the data by individual disability categories. At the same time, the term "able-bodied" is also misleading, since it includes an equally heterogeneous group in terms of age, sex and actual physical well-being. Second, in comparing the disabled and able-bodied groups, no attempt was made to match them for age, sex and other parameters which would make it possible to isolate and study more directly the effect of the physical status variable. Thus, although the comparison is based on physical status, this does not imply that any differences identified between the two groups represent a causal relationship between physical status and a particular finding. Nonetheless, the trends are suggestive of such a relationship and are consistent with the findings of others. For example, Sadoughi et al.[11] reported a decline in sexual activity by 78 per cent of 55 patients after the onset of a chronic disability. Third, the data reported here were obtained through anonymous questionnaires. Although every effort was made to maintain confidentiality, there are still all the problems and limitations associated with questionnaire data inherent in the results. And fourth, persons who attended the workshops represent a highly motivated and self-selected group which makes generalization or comparisons with other groups difficult (with the possible exception of other SAR program participants).

With these constraints in mind, there are still a number of useful insights and preliminary conclusions that can be drawn with regard to this population of SAR participants and the two major subgroups studied. In the area of attitude change, the results indicate the able-bodied participants experienced more change toward increased comfort than did the disabled participants as a result of attending the workshop. The disabled group experienced most change with behaviors that are considered less anxiety provoking such as masturbation and heterosexual activity, while both groups experienced least change with group sex, which is still somewhat taboo and therefore likely to produce greater discomfort. These findings tend to dispute the notion that disabled persons are more comfortable with sexuality in general because they have had to deal with it more openly.

In terms of sexual experience, there was not a large difference for behaviors-ever-tried between the two groups. Although the numbers are small and should not be overinterpreted, the greater homosexuality experience among the disabled group is of interest and may reflect an increased willingness and/or need to explore homosexual inclinations because of decreased opportunities in a heterosexual context.

The most significant differences in sexual behavior between the two groups, as one might expect, were revealed in an analysis of experience over the six months preceding the workshop. With the exception of homosexuality, experience rates were one-third less in the disabled group with virtually no difference in the level of activity for any one behavior. Regardless of the level of activity, however, it is of interest that both groups expressed similarly high levels of dissatisfaction and listed the same three problems among the top five as reasons for their dissatisfaction. Although the population and methods are not directly comparable, these findings are in contrast to those of Sadoughi and co-workers in the study cited earlier.[11] In her study, only 36 per cent of persons with a chronic disability expressed a desire for more satisfaction in their current sexual activity, and disability-related limitations were the most frequently mentioned reasons for feelings of discomfort in carrying out sexual activity. With regard to activity levels of specific sexual behaviors, most reports tend to stress physiological functioning such as erections, ejaculation and orgasm and do not distinguish between current activity and behaviors ever experienced.[12-14] The one exception to this is coitus which has been investigated by a number of authors primarily in persons with spinal cord injury. Zeitlin et al.[15] reported that 20 per cent of 100 spinal cord injured men had experienced penile-vaginal intercourse. Among 150 patients studied by Comarr,[16] 38 per cent reported attempting it but only 24 per cent of those stated they were successful. In another study by Comarr,[17] he called attention to the relation of the level and completeness of a spinal injury to sexual functioning. Among patients who attempted sexual intercourse, success rates ranged from 65 per cent for persons with complete lower motor neuron lesions to 90 per cent for those with incomplete lower motor neuron lesions. Finally, in a group of 31 spinal cord injured women, Bregman and Hadley[18] found that 90 per cent had experienced intercourse since their injury.

SECTION IV: **Impact of the SAR Program**

Although TIRR is closely affiliated with Baylor College of Medicine, the program was not sponsored or funded by the medical school. Rather, the program was initiated by hospital staff as a volunteer effort to fulfill unmet needs of both patients and staff. Because of the cultural and social climate associated with this region of the country, we elected to maintain a low profile and build slowly from within our own institution. In retrospect, this appears to have been a sound decision. Although there may have been more flexibility and space if the workshops had been held in an outside facility, there would have been the disadvantages of greater overhead, possible financial insolvency and probable adverse response from the community. However, the greatest disadvantage would have been the risk of isolating the program from the hospital which would have minimized its visibility and impact on the rest of the Institute. As a result of remaining highly visible both physically and psychologically, the SAR workshops have helped catalyze a number of additional activities dealing with human sexuality elsewhere in the hospital. Together these efforts have helped legitimize sexuality as a basic health care right that should be dealt with as part of a comprehensive rehabilitation program.

In a recent survey of hospital employees, 172 or 89 per cent of those responding agreed that the rehabilitation staff should help patients with sexual problems and adjustments. Only 3 per cent said they should not and 8 per cent said they were uncertain. In response to the question, "Who should provide help in the area of sexuality?" 63 per cent said the whole team, 29 per cent said physicians, 28 per cent said social workers, and 18 per cent said nurses. Although there are no data which indicate how many members of the staff actually discuss sexual matters with each patient, it is clear that an increasingly large number of the staff are sensitized to the general area and feel more comfortable talking about the topic.

It has been our conviction from the beginning of the program, that the problems of sexuality did not belong exclusively to one discipline. This is especially pertinent in rehabilitation, where a number of disciplines are involved in providing comprehensive care. Rehabilitation traditionally uses a coordinated team approach to assist the patient in regaining the maximum possible function in activities of daily living and all psychosocial-vocational areas. It is logical then that sexuality should be viewed as an area in which all members of the team can make a contribution—from providing factual information to helping a patient feel more comfortable in asking questions and bringing anxieties and feelings to the surface.

This growing hospital-wide concern with the importance of sexuality is reflected in other ways as well. Table 14 shows the number of staff

Table 14. Staff Volunteers By Discipline For 1974

Discipline	Number
Nursing	10
Physical Therapy	9
Social Service	9
Medicine	6
Occupational Therapy	4
Photography	4
Secretary	4
Miscellaneous (6)	6
Total	52
Total number of disciplines represented	13

volunteers by discipline during 1974. Fifty-two persons representing 13 disciplines volunteered time to help with the many tasks which make the program possible. This sizeable volunteer staff make the human sexuality program the single largest ongoing interdisciplinary activity in the hospital.

As a consequence of this heightened interest and concern with sexuality as part of the rehabilitative process, there have been repeated requests for additional information and services which have provided the stimulus for generating new activities and programs in various parts of the hospital. During 1974, weekly rap sessions called "Sex and Coffee" were initiated for inpatients and their significant others.[19] These are led by a physician and social worker and include selected films from the workshop, educational materials and informal discussion. Similar kinds of educational-counseling sessions have been initiated in other hospitals as part of a larger program in human sexuality. These include the efforts of Romano and Lassiter[20] in Ann Arbor, Michigan, Miller et al.[21] in Columbus, Ohio, and Eisenberg and Rustad[22] in Cleveland. In 1975, a comprehensive sexual inventory of 120 questions was developed at TIRR to provide more specific information concerning the problems and techniques of sexual adjustment. This questionnaire was designed in a multidisciplinary effort by physicians, nurses, social workers and physical therapists and is being administered to discharged spinal cord injured adults. It was developed in direct response to our finding that a majority of the disabled workshop participants were sexually unsatisfied, and we as professionals had inadequate information to answer many of their specific questions and needs. Finally, during 1976 a collaborative effort by a group of basic scientists and clinicians was initiated to investigate more fully the residual neurophysiological sexual function in male patients with spinal cord injuries and to explore possible therapeutic techniques for enhancing that function.[23]

In addition to the tangible impact of the SAR program on the Institute and its staff, there has been an equally important if less tangible impact on the community. For many of the participants, it was their first visit inside the Institute and often their first exposure to the field of rehabilitation. Based on written and informal comments, it is clear that this kind of workshop, which brings the able-bodied and handicapped together to share and learn from each other, provides a powerful tool for educating the public regarding the promise and accomplishments of rehabilitation.

SECTION V: **Conclusion**

These findings have a number of implications with regard to sexual counseling and areas for further research. First, as Diamond[24] and others have pointed out, it is clear that many of the principles of sexual counseling apply equally to disabled and able-bodied persons—i.e., the importance of the partners' total relationship, the need for good communication and the willingness to experiment as a way of sustaining sexual interest. Second, handicap-related problems play a sizeable role in decreasing sexual activity among the disabled. In the group studied here, 36 per cent implicated a physical problem as one of the major reasons for diminished sexual activity. In general, however, most of these problems cannot be resolved with counseling intervention alone. Difficulties cited most frequently were spasticity, pain and an inability to sustain an erection—none of which is easily resolved or ameliorated by current medical or surgical techniques. What is required is an interdisciplinary research effort to gain a better understanding of the underlying organic and psychologic mechanisms which result in specific sexual dysfunctions. Satisfactory management will then, in turn, depend upon an interdisciplinary team approach. One such effort with regard to impotence in spinal cord injury is already underway by Halstead, Karacan and co-workers.[23,25] Finally, there is the problem of lack of partners which was the most common reason for decreased sexual activity in both groups. In response to this need, it is our feeling that surrogates offer an important and under-utilized therapeutic option initially, but in the long run can only play a limited role. In addition to the legal issues associated with the use of surrogates in this country, surrogate relationships fail to provide the deeper need most people have for a longer-term emotional commitment.

Despite the significant progress made in expanding our efforts in the area of sexuality over the past four years, there are still a number of problems that remain unsolved. One of the biggest of these is patient financing. Approximately 16 per cent of the patients who attended workshops were sponsored by third-party payers, while the remainder either received scholarships or paid the tuition themselves ($25 for patients). Until we are more successful in convincing all rehabilitation sponsors that sexuality is a basic health care right, the financial barrier will continue to deny a sizeable number of clients this service. A second problem is the lack of adequate counseling and therapy services. Many of the patients who complete the hospital rehabilitation program and attend the workshops are still in need of ongoing sexual counseling and support. At the present time, both the Institute's and the community's resources in these areas are limited, even for those who can afford them. In our experience, this is one of the unfortunate ironies of the SAR workshops: they have helped create a demand for services that don't always exist. In many ways, meeting this demand is now the biggest challenge which lies ahead.

Others have identified a number of additional unanswered questions that have been posed as a result of our raised consciousness regarding sexuality among the disabled. Griffith et al.[26] in a review of the literature up to 1973 pertaining to sexual function in spinal cord injured patients identified five areas that deserve further investigation. These include 1) attitudes and feelings of both sexual partners toward their relationship and its physical expressions; 2) mechanical aspects of sexual activities including kinesiology, physiology, alternate sexual behaviors and adaptive devices; 3) up-to-date endocrinologic information; 4) measurements of effectiveness of methods of modifying attitudes and increasing information and skills of those health professionals counseling these patients; and 5) systems of analysis of methods of evaluation and treatment. More recently, in a review of the psychosocial considerations of sexuality and SCI, Teal and Athelstan[27] conclude that despite a number of articles dealing with this area, there are still substantial needs for well-designed, sound research efforts to increase our knowledge base.

REFERENCES

1. Weiss, A.J. and Diamond, M.D. Sexual adjustment, identification, and attitudes of patients with myelopathy. Arch. Phys. Med. Rehab. 245, 1966.
2. Richardson, S.A. People with Cerebral Palsy Talk for Themselves. In Rubinstein, E.A. et al. (Eds.) New Directions in Sex Research. New York, Plenum Press, 1976.
3. Cole, T.M. Sexuality and physical disabilities. Arch. Sex. Behav. 4:389, 1975.
4. Ayres, T. et al. SARguide for a Better Sex Life. San Francisco, The National Sex Forum, 1975. (L.C. No. 75-7218, ISBN 0-913566-01-2)
5. Chilgren, R.A. and Briggs, M.M. On being explicit: sex education for professionals. SIECUS Report 1:1, 1973.
6. Cole, T.M. et al. New program of sex education and counseling for spinal cord injured adults and health care professionals. Int. J. Paraplegia 11:111, 1973.
7. Halstead, L.S. et al. An interdisciplinary program on human sexuality for health care professionals and the physically disabled. South. Med. J. 69:1352, 1976.
8. Halstead, L.S. et al. A hospital-based program in human sexuality. Arch. Phys. Med. Rehabil. 58:409, 1977.
9. Held, J.P. et al. Sexual attitude reassessment workshops: effect on spinal cord injured adults, their partners and rehabilitation professionals. Arch. Phys. Med. Rehabil. 56:14, 1975.
10. Cole, T.M. Sexuality and the Physically Handicapped. In Green, R. (Ed.) Human Sexuality: A Health Practitioner's Text. Baltimore, Williams and Wilkins, 1975.
11. Sadoughi, S. et al. Sexual adjustment in a chronically ill and physically disabled population: A pilot study. Arch. Phys. Med. Rehabil. 52:311, 1971.
12. Munro, D. et al. Effect of injury to spinal cord and cauda equina on sexual potency of men. N. Engl. J. Med. 239:903, 1948.
13. Talbot, H.S. Report on sexual function in paraplegics. J. Urol. 61:265, 1949.
14. Talbot, H.S. Sexual function in paraplegia. J. Urol. 73:91, 1955.
15. Zeitlin, A.B. et al. Sexology of paraplegic male. Fertil. Steril. 8:337, 1957.
16. Comarr, A.E. Sexual function among patients with spinal cord injury. Urol. Int. 25:134, 1970.
17. Comarr, A.E. Sexual concepts in traumatic cord and cauda equina lesions. J. Urol. 106:375, 1971.
18. Bregman, S. and Hadley, R.G. Sexual adjustment and feminine attractiveness among spinal cord injured women. Arch. Phys. Med. Rehabil. 57:448, 1976.
19. Holden, B.L. and Meier, R.H. Sex and coffee: A sexual counseling approach. Presented at the American Congress of Rehabilitation Medicine Annual Meeting, 52nd Session, Atlanta, Nov., 1975.
20. Romano, M.D. and Lassiter, R.E. Sexual counseling with spinal cord injured. Arch. Phys. Med. Rehab. 53:568, 1972.
21. Miller, D.K. et al. Therapeutic groups for patients with spinal cord injuries. Arch. Phys. Med. Rehab. 56:130, 1975.
22. Eisenberg, M.G. and Rustad, L.C. Sex education and counseling program on a spinal cord injury service. Arch. Phys. Med. Rehab. 57:135, 1976.

23. Halstead, L.S. et al. Impotence in Spinal Cord Injury: Evaluation, Diagnosis and Management. Paper presented at the Texas Medical Assoc. Annual Meeting, Houston, May, 1977.
24. Diamond, M. Sexuality and the handicapped. Rehabil. Lit. 35:34, 1974.
25. Karacan, I. et al. Nocturnal Penile Tumescence (NPT) and Sleep Stages in Patients with Spinal Cord Injuries. Paper presented at the International Sleep Research Assoc. Annual Meeting, Houston, April, 1977.
26. Griffith, E.R. et al. Sexual function in spinal cord-injured patients: A review. Arch. Phys. Med. Rehab. 54:539, 1973.
27. Teal, J.C. and Athelstan, G.T. Sexuality and spinal cord injury: Some psychosocial considerations. Arch. Phys. Med. Rehabil. 56:264, 1975.

23

Sexual Disability in
Congenital Syndromes

Use of Phallometry in Erectile Dysfunction

ALEX COMFORT, M.B.

Many congenital disorders have obvious practical effects on the sexuality of their possessors if they affect motor and sensory function, liability to injury (hemophilia, fragilitas ossium), deformity and unusual appearance (achondroplasia, albinism), or ease of delivery in women, or if they entail extensive preventive surgery (premalignant intestinal polyposis). Conditions involving sex chromatin or apparent gender are recognized by the physician as sexual, and adjustment is usually attempted; reference should be made to the extensive literature of these disorders. The cases where sexual problems are most likely to be missed are those not frankly involving the genitalia, where other problems overshadow the effect of the disability on the sexual life of the patient.

In all cases of impaired function or unusual susceptibility or appearance, sexual problems should be addressed by direct inquiry. Any disability which impairs movement, affects joints or muscles, alters the patient's conformity to the cultural ideal of sexual desirability, produces dyspnea on moderate exertion, or affects the likely expectation of life and the amount of time which must be spent in precautions or treatment will have physical or psychical effects on sexual self-image, performance or both. These must be dealt with on an individual basis by inquiry, imaginative thought, and improvisation. There is very little documentation either of specific sexual effects in uncommoner disorders, or of their management in either sex, and no substitute for frank inquiry from patients, including patients who have devised ways of coping. The physician who wants to know if and how Marfan's syndrome, for instance, affects sexual activity can find out only by consulting patients. Obstetric hazards, e.g., in achondroplasia, are well-documented by contrast. In general the physical consequences of common problems (muscular dystrophies, for example) in the male, and of *all* unusual states of health or physiology in women, are very poorly covered in textbooks and in the literature.

As with all the disabled, people subject to constitutional health problems suffer both the effects of those problems on physiology and the psychical consequences of unusualness, extended medication and anxiety about injury, prognosis and physical appearance. These may be compounded by genetic problems concerning reproduction and the transmission of heritable syndromes to offspring. *All* of these responses of the patient require imaginative approaches as part of the treatment of the underlying condition. In this respect, congenital abnormalities are not unique, but the patient with acquired asthma reacts differently regarding sexual disability compared with the patient whose problem has been lifelong and whose expectations have been moulded by it. Interference with sexuality should not be described as a feature of a syndrome without allowance being made for general factors, such as the chronic expectation of invalidism and the time spent in the hospital or for special treatment. At the same time, objective data of interest on sexual function in several rare disorders (familial dysautonomia, for example) have rarely been collected.

The management of sexual problems in congenitally exceptional individuals involves 1) *inquiry*: ascertain what the patient can and cannot do, and the exact nature of any impairment. This may range from paralysis or erectile incompetence to painful interference by an exostosis, and from dyspnea in intercourse to fear of pregnancy; 2) *objective testing* of sexual function by sleep phallometry in men and measurement of lubrication in women before nonfunction is assumed to be biochemical or neural in origin; 3) *strategy planning* to circumvent specific problems such as stiffness or liability to injury; 4) *rehabilitation* in which the patient's realistic options are explored, anxieties are dealt with, and sexuality is viewed as part of the general problem of living with disability while avoiding career invalidism. All of these interventions should be begun as early as possible, so as to avoid bewitchment by diagnosis and ensure that the patient's view of sexual, as of other, options, is realistic. Sexual activity has been traditionally regarded as magically dangerous in this culture, and for this reason it may be a particular anxiety to people who need to "be careful," either following a heart attack or by reason of constitutional vulnerability. Such anxiety may itself also represent a *nolo contendere,* when self-image is impaired. Non-involvement in sex, as in other activities, must be a patient choice, but the choice should be discussed and thus informed.

In regard to the effects of appearance on self-valuation, people differ enormously. Most achondroplastics, for example, accommodate to their disability—achondroplastic women are often happily married in spite of the added obstetrical difficulty. In other kinds of unusual appearance the choice has to be made between acceptance and concealment. Extensive plastic surgery can be justified, e.g., in hypertelorism, provided the patient has a realistic idea of the outcome. It is more to the point to let such a patient talk beforehand to a happily married person with the same problem who has not had surgery, and then decide if the exercise is worthwhile. It should be remembered that sources of self-value are perhaps the most important single quantity in psychiatry; the congenitally exceptional person needs to develop a "set" in which self-value is compatible with the real condition and is invulnerable to rejection by the uninformed, and sexual rehabilitation can be an important part of this process. It is an important unspoken part of any request for surgery—"so that I can be more active" or "so that I can do as others do."

Both in counseling the congenitally disabled and in general sex counseling, it pays to remember that lack of libido, lack of orgasm, and lack of erection are more often attitudinal than physical, can be iatrogenic, and are rarely endocrinal unless the endocrine deficit is obvious. At the same time, renewed awareness that this is so sometimes leads to missing either a physical effect or the mechanism by which sexual anxiety is being mediated, e.g., non-ejaculation. Objective measurement has become easier with increased patient frankness (see PHALLOMETRY) and should be performed if there is doubt, and before embarking on extensive psychotherapy or telling the patient that "nothing can be done." Sexual response can now be investigated by other than the traditional anecdotal approach, and where biochemical or neural problems are suspected, it must be investigated.

For congenital endocrine syndromes, reference should be made to a textbook on that subject. Although low sexual drive in women is not a "congenital syndrome" as far as we know, reference is made to it here to illustrate a general difficulty: androgen levels in sexually anesthetic women are often low, but inhibition of arousal almost certainly itself affects gonadotrophin release, so that a chicken-and-egg phenomenon exists. History of anorgasmia in a mother and sisters might be evidence of other than physical causation as readily as of "heritable defect."

Hormonal control of libido is distinct from hormonal control of sexual function. In the female it is almost certainly mediated by androgen and is increased experimentally when androgen is administered. In males androgen may or may not affect libido, or appear to do so: increased LH and androgen levels appear to be the result, rather than the cause, of libidinal increase. It is arguable that if they both increased it, and were increased by it, a positive feedback would exist. However in congenital defect of LHRH and LH production, libido is absent although spermatogenesis is normal.

Androgen-induced hypersexuality in women does not appear to have a male counterpart. Male hypersexuality is rarely complained of. The possibility that libido in males might be controlled by some other LH-released substance, not testosterone, is negated by the absence of hypersexuality in the testicular feminization syndrome, where tissue insensitivity to testosterone produces LH overdrive. There is no evidence that the FSH-tubulin system involved in spermatogenesis has any part in mediating arousal. Accordingly, the reported, and fairly consistent, erotization of low-drive males by HCG might be inferred to be (a) a placebo effect—readily induced in this area; (b) the result of the presence of a material other than FSH and LH in the extract; (c) the result of a higher local production of androgen at the Leydig cell than can be reliably produced by androgen administration. In many cases non-response is due to frankly inadequate dosage.[1]

It is possible that definite evidence of endocrine hypersexuality in men may have been missed for cultural reasons. It might well be looked for in known neuroendocrine syndromes where sexual responsiveness has so far been scored as normal. LH levels in men appear to rise slowly with aging at a time when sexual response-speed declines; this is in line with their control by androgen. The complexity of this system should discourage indiscriminate use of, and claims for, androgen as a resexualizing agent where low libido is not associated with demonstrably low androgen levels and high levels of free binding-protein. There are relatively few non-endocrine syndromes associated with specific disability where this is the case.

REFERENCE

1. Greenblatt, R.B. *in* Freedman, A.M., Kaplan, H.I. and Sadock, B.J. (Eds.) Comprehensive Textbook of Psychiatry. Baltimore, Williams and Wilkins (2nd Ed.), 1975, p. 1383.

PHALLOMETRY IN ERECTILE DYSFUNCTION

Phallometry during REM sleep and by direct measurement of the unerect and erect penis, supplemented by standardized photography, should form part of the investigation of any organic or intractable erectile difficulty. *Sleep phallometry* tests the integrity of the erectile mechanism: in psychogenic impotence erection will be normal. The method used is that described by Karacan et al.[1,4-6] using strain-gauges at the coronal sulcus and penis root. A simultaneous EEG is required to establish REM sleep. In normal males, erection will be observed during periods totaling about 100 minutes per night's sleep. Drugs affecting REM sleep (including MAO inhibitors, alcohol and many sedatives) must be suitably withdrawn for the test.

Waking phallometry may be used in cases where erection occurs but is in some way inadequate. It can be done by direct measurement and may if necessary be left to the instructed patient. An increase of 16–20 mm. in basal shaft circumference usually indicates adequate erection. This is 1½ to 3 times greater than the coronal change. In Peyronie's disease, or in any other interference with the distribution of blood in the corpora, this ratio may be disturbed or reversed, leading to a soft or collapsible erection. *Photography* is invaluable in pinpointing the precise change. It also shows the pre-ejaculatory engorgement of the glans which belongs to the "phase of inevitability" and is usually not seen in REM sleep erection, where no emission occurs. Age, and certain drugs, notably MAO inhibitors, tricyclics and phenothiazines, inhibit this change when they produce non-ejaculation or delayed ejaculation, but usually not when ejaculation is retrograde.

Adequate filling of the shaft and at the sulcus with relative flaccidity of the glans is common in so-called ejaculatory incapacity. In premature ejaculation the glans may become tense before the corpora have entirely filled. This is difficult to observe, since premature ejaculation is less common during masturbation, but it may be detected photographically. The non-filled glans has a dull surface which becomes shiny only at the moment of complete distension. Preclimactic filling is probably part of the ejaculatory, not the erectile, reflex, and may depend on the initial muscle spasms which precede orgasm, since it can be simulated by pressure over the perineum.

If failure of penetration is a complaint, penile rigidity and stability should be tested by pressure against a standard thin rubber diaphragm. A penis may be unstable even with firm erection if its basal insertion is abnormal congenitally or as a result of trauma. For this and many other reasons, complaints of failing erection or selective impotence should not automatically be taken as psychogenic. They commonly are, but

PHALLOMETRY

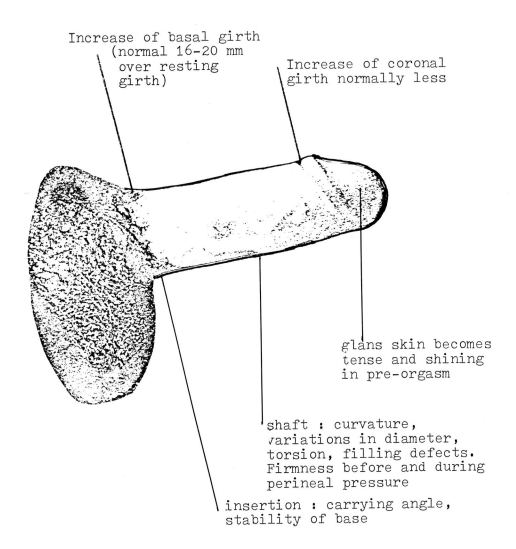

Increase of basal girth
(normal 16-20 mm
over resting
girth)

Increase of coronal
girth normally less

glans skin becomes
tense and shining
in pre-orgasm

shaft : curvature,
variations in diameter,
torsion, filling defects.
Firmness before and during
perineal pressure

insertion : carrying angle,
stability of base

PHOTOGRAPHY

mechanical defects also occur and can only be identified by proper examination. *Careful history,* including a full inquiry into what the patient actually experiences, should be combined with *examination of the
partner* wherever possible, since women differ appreciably in the ease
with which they are penetrated in the most common coital position.

In regard to erectile-ejaculatory difficulties due to drugs or to disease,
standardization of these findings has only recently begun, but inspection,

either of an erection or of photographs if the patient is embarrassed, enables the urologist or the physician to see what is occurring—i.e., whether the failure is global, affects the filling of the shaft, affects the stability of the erect organ, or involves the ejaculatory reflex and its precursors.

Sleep phallometry is more time-consuming and more expensive but clearly establishes the extent of a psychogenic component and is mandatory before any consideration of prosthetic surgery. The desirability of doing sleep phallometry before elective prostatectomy has to be offset against the risk of creating impotence by suggestion. Done properly as an element in active sexual rehabilitation, it could well have a positive effect. It is also mandatory in any case of impotence which does not respond fairly rapidly to reassurance and psychotherapy; much time can be wasted on the psychotherapy of an undiagnosed Peyronie's disease, and much can be gained by a clear demonstration to the patient that the erectile mechanism is in order. A urological or sexological department dealing in male problems should be routinely able to undertake the investigations here described.

BIBLIOGRAPHY

1. Karacan, I. A simple and inexpensive transducer for quantitative measurements of penile erection during sleep. Behav. Res. Math. Instrum. 1:251, 1969.
2. _____, Goodenough, D.R., Shapiro, R. and Starker, S. Erection during sleep in its relation to dream anxiety. Arch. Gen. Psychiat. 15:183, 1966.
3. _____, Scott, F.B., Gross, J. and Zuch, J. Cycle of penile erection synchronous with dreaming (REM) sleep. Arch. Gen. Psychiat. 12:29.
4. _____, Williams, R.L., Thornby, J.I. and Salis, P.J. Sleep related tumescence as a function of age. Amer. J. Psychiat. 132:932, 1975.
5. _____, Scott, et al. Nocturnal erections, differential diagnosis of impotence, and diabetes. Biol. Psychiat. 12:373, 1977.
6. _____. Advances in the diagnosis of erectile impotence. Med. Asp. Hum. Sexual. 12:85, 1978.

Index

Numerals in *italics* indicate figures or tables.

284

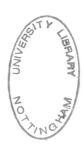